High Protein Cookbook For Seniors

Quick and Easy Delicious Meals For Healthy Aging

Dr. Josephine S. Sanger

Table of Content

Nutrition plays a crucial role in the general

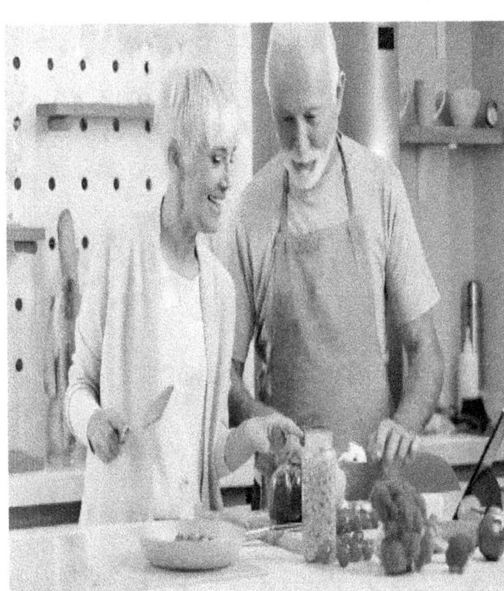

health and well-being of seniors. As we age, Our bodies experience changes that affect nutrient absorption, metabolism, and overall nutritional requirements. A well-balanced and nutrient-dense diet becomes increasingly vital to support aging bodies and keep optimal health. Proper nutrition for seniors adds to the following:

★ ***Disease Prevention:*** A nutritious diet can help avoid or manage various chronic conditions common in older adults, such as heart disease, diabetes, and osteoporosis.

★ ***Immune Function:*** Adequate nutrition supports a robust immune system, helping seniors avoid infections and diseases.

★ ***Energy Levels:*** Proper nutrients provide the energy needed for daily activities, supporting independence and an active lifestyle.

★ ***Cognitive Health:*** Certain nutrients, like omega-3 fatty acids and antioxidants, play a role in maintaining cognitive function and lowering the risk of cognitive decline.

★ ***Bone Health:*** Calcium and vitamin D are important for maintaining bone health and preventing osteoporosis, a condition prevalent in aging populations.

Overview of High Protein Diets:

High-protein diets are characterized by an increased intake of protein-rich foods, stressing their benefits for various aspects of health. In the setting of seniors, a high-protein diet offers several advantages:

➤ ***Muscle Preservation:*** Aging often leads to muscle loss, but a high protein diet can help maintain muscle mass, promoting strength and avoiding frailty.

➢ *Weight Management:* Protein-rich foods provide a feeling of satiety, helping seniors maintain a healthy weight by reducing the chance of overeating.

➢ *Metabolic Health:* Protein plays a part in regulating metabolism, which becomes especially important as the metabolic rate tends to decrease with age.

➢ *Blood Sugar Control:* Adequate protein intake can help in stabilizing blood sugar levels, beneficial for seniors managing or preventing diabetes.

Introduction

Welcome to "High Protein Diet Cookbook for Seniors" – a comprehensive guide crafted to empower the golden years with the incredible potential of nutrition.

Aging gracefully begins with nourishing your body, and this cookbook is your compass to a vibrant and healthy life. In these pages, we embark on a journey that transcends mere recipes, diving into the transformative power of food as medicine.

As we age, the significance of a well-balanced diet, rich in proteins, becomes paramount. This cookbook is not just a collection of delicious recipes; it's a testament to the profound impact food choices have on preventing diseases and enhancing overall well-being. From understanding the unique nutritional needs of seniors to mastering the art of meal preparation, each chapter unfolds a wealth of knowledge.

Explore a diverse array of protein-rich foods, learn cooking techniques that preserve nutrients, and discover the joy of crafting meals that nourish both body and soul.

With easy-to-follow recipes, helpful tips, and a focus on superfoods, this cookbook is your companion on the path to a healthier, more fulfilling senior life. Welcome to a journey where food becomes not just sustenance but a celebration of vitality!

Chapter 1: Understanding Senior Diets and Nutrients

Nutritional Needs of Seniors: As people age, their nutritional needs change due to factors such as altered metabolism, reduced energy expenditure, and changes in body composition. Understanding the specific nutritional needs of seniors is important for keeping health and well-being. Key factors include:

- ***Protein:*** Seniors often require more protein to counteract muscle loss, support immune function, and keep overall health.
- ***Fiber:*** Promotes digestive health, prevents constipation, and supports heart health.

- *Vitamin B12:* Important for nerve function and red blood cell production, as absorption drops with age.

- *Potassium:* Helps keep blood pressure and electrolyte balance.

- *Omega-3 Fatty Acids:* Support heart health and may help cognitive function.

Common Health Concerns for Seniors:

★ *Cardiovascular Disease:* Increases in prevalence with age, making heart health a major concern.

★ *Osteoporosis:* Bone density decreases, leading to a greater chance of fractures.

★ ***Diabetes:*** Prevalence grows, necessitating careful management of blood sugar levels.

★ ***Arthritis:*** Joint health becomes a worry, impacting mobility and daily activities.

★ ***Cognitive Decline:*** Age-related cognitive conditions, such as Alzheimer's disease, become more common.

★ ***Vision and Hearing Issues:*** Sensory impairments can affect freedom and quality of life.

★ ***Immune System Weakness:*** Aging compromises immune function, making seniors more open to infections.

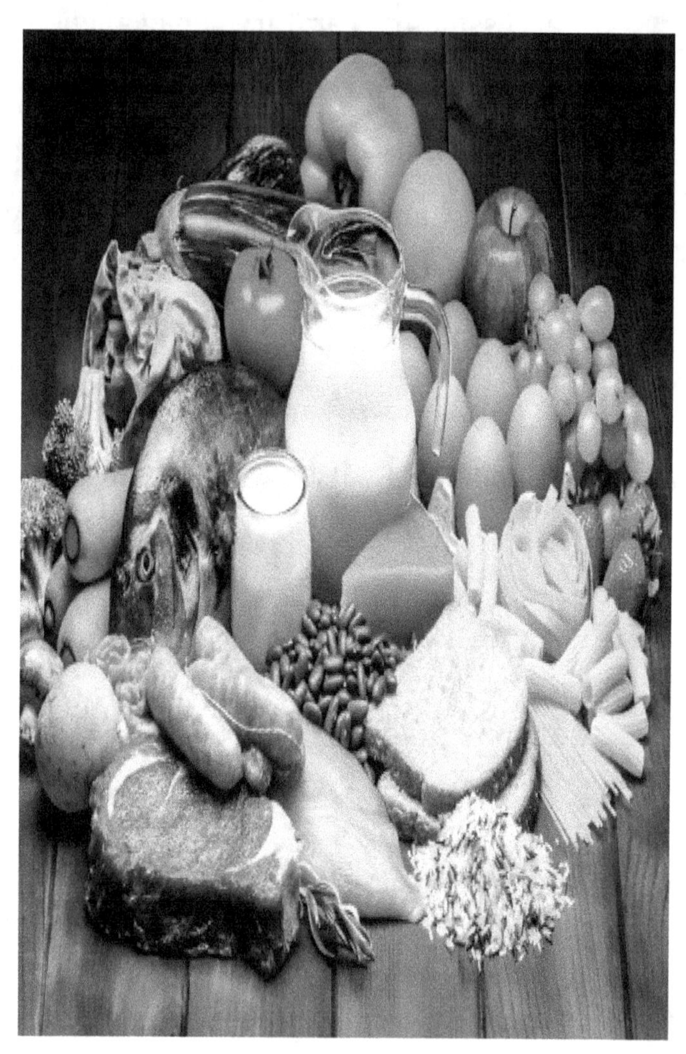

Chapter 2: Building a Healthy Plate for High-Protein Diets for Seniors

Constructing a healthy plate for seniors involves balancing macronutrients, with a particular focus on incorporating sufficient protein. Here's a breakdown:

> ***Protein-Rich Foods:*** Select high-quality protein sources such as lean meats, poultry, fish, eggs, dairy, legumes, and plant-based proteins. This ensures an adequate intake of important amino acids crucial for muscle maintenance.

> ***Colorful veggies and Fruits:*** Fill a portion of the plate with a variety of colorful veggies and fruits. These provide important vitamins, minerals, antioxidants, and dietary fiber,

supporting overall health and digestion.

➤ ***Whole Grains:*** Include a dish of whole grains like brown rice, quinoa, or whole-grain bread. Whole grains offer complex carbohydrates, fiber, and additional nutrients, adding to sustained energy levels and promoting digestive health.

➤ ***Healthy Fats:*** Incorporate sources of healthy fats, such as avocados, nuts, seeds, and olive oil, in balance. These fats add to satiety, support nutrient absorption, and provide essential fatty acids.

➤ ***Dairy or Dairy Alternatives:*** Include a serving of dairy or fortified dairy alternatives to ensure a proper calcium and vitamin D intake for bone health.

➤ **Hydration:** Accompany the meal with water or other low-calorie beverages to stay properly hydrated. Proper hydration is important for digestion, kidney function, and overall well-being.

Meal Planning for High-Protein Diets for Seniors:

Effective meal planning for seniors on high-protein diets involves careful consideration of nutritional needs, preferences, and practicality:

- Diverse Protein Sources: Plan meals that include a variety of protein sources to ensure a broad spectrum of necessary amino acids. This could include rotating between different types of meats, adding plant-based proteins, and utilizing dairy or dairy alternatives.

- Balanced Nutrient Intake: Ensure a mix of macronutrients (protein, carbohydrates, and fats) along with an array of vitamins and minerals. This supports overall health and addresses specific nutritional needs linked with aging.

- Portion Control: Consider portion sizes to meet individual energy needs and prevent overeating. Adjust portions based on things such as activity level, metabolic rate, and health conditions.

- Regular, Balanced Meals: Aim for regular meals throughout the day to keep consistent energy levels and support optimal metabolism. Include protein-rich snacks if needed to meet daily protein goals.

- Variety in Cooking Techniques: Explore different cooking methods to improve flavors without compromising nutritional value. Grilling, baking, steaming, and sautéing are healthy choices that retain nutrients in the food.

- Incorporate Superfoods: Integrate nutrient-dense superfoods into meals to improve health benefits. Examples include berries, fresh greens, nuts, seeds, and fatty fish rich in omega-3 fatty acids.

- ❖ Salmon: A fatty fish rich in omega-3 fatty acids and high-quality protein, supporting heart health and muscle repair.

- ❖ Chicken Breast: Lean and versatile, chicken breast is an excellent source of protein for seniors, helping in muscle preservation.

- ❖ Greek Yogurt: Packed with protein and probiotics, Greek yogurt is beneficial for digestive health and provides important nutrients like calcium.

- ❖ Eggs: A complete protein source containing all essential amino acids, eggs add to muscle health and overall nutrition.

- ❖ Quinoa: A whole grain that is also a full protein, quinoa is rich in fiber, vitamins, and minerals.

- ❖ Cottage Cheese: High in protein and low in fat, cottage cheese is a handy and versatile ingredient for seniors.

- ❖ Beans and Legumes: Lentils, chickpeas, and black beans are protein-rich plant-based options that also provide fiber and other important nutrients.

- ❖ Tofu: A plant-based protein source made from soybeans, tofu is versatile and can be incorporated into different dishes.

- ❖ Lean Beef: A good source of high-quality protein, lean cuts of beef also provide important nutrients like iron and zinc.

❖ Nuts and Seeds: Almonds, walnuts, chia seeds, and flaxseeds are nutrient-dense sources of protein, healthy fats, and vitamins.

7-Day Meal Plan:

Day 1:

- **Breakfast:** Tuna Noodle Casserole
- **Lunch:** Rainbow Quinoa Salad
- **Dinner:** Lamb Chop with Sweet Potato Mash & Vegetables

Day 2:

- **Breakfast:** Muesli with Yoghurt & Fruit
- **Lunch:** Chicken Salad with Flatbread

- *Dinner:* Bulgur Wheat salad With poached Egg

Day 3:

- *Breakfast:* frittata with Cottage Cheese and Vegetables
- *Lunch:* Tuna & Avocado Salad on Toast
- *Dinner:* Beef & Black Bean stir-fry with Rice Noodles

Day 4:

- *Breakfast:* Coconut and Blueberry baked oats
- *Lunch:* Chickpea & Barley Salad
- *Dinner:* Spaghetti Bolognese

<u>*Day 5:*</u>

- ***Breakfast:*** Porridge with Fruit
- ***Lunch:*** Chicken & Pasta Salad
- ***Dinner:*** Spaghetti Bolognese

<u>*Day 6:*</u>

- ***Breakfast:*** Banana & Chocolate Smoothie
- ***Lunch:*** Spiced Sweet Potato and Chickpea Fritters with Soft Boiled Eggs
- ***Dinner:*** Pork Chops & Vegetables

<u>*Day 7:*</u>

- ***Breakfast:*** Omelet with Vegetables
- ***Lunch:*** Beef & Noodle Lettuce Cups

- ***Dinner:*** Grilled Chicken with Rice & Vegetable Salad

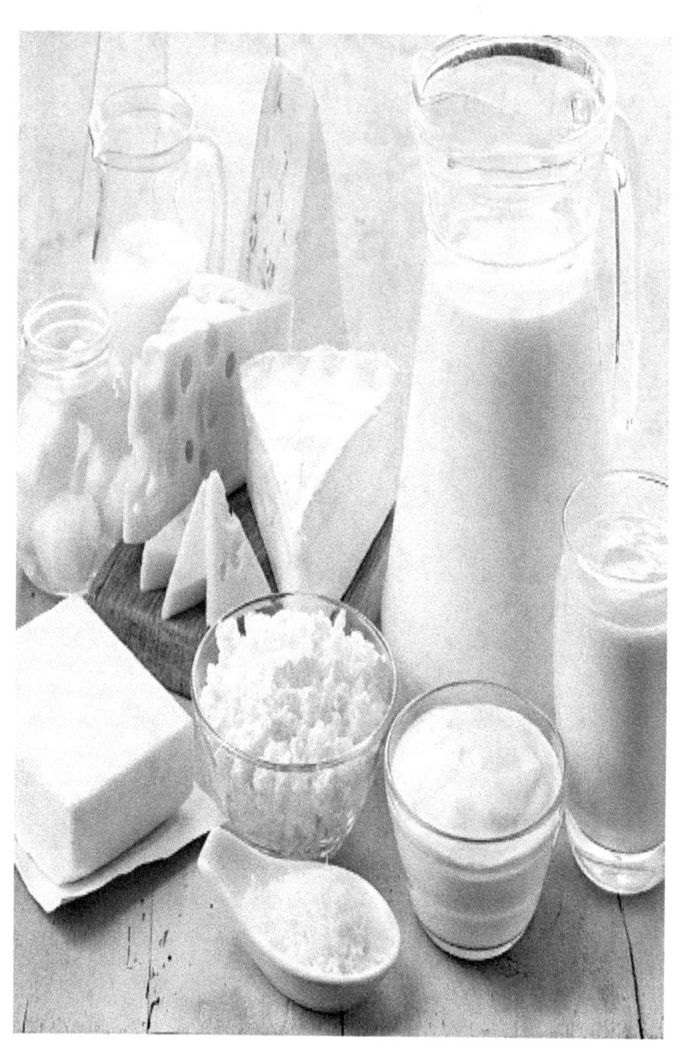

Chapter 3: High-Protein Recipes

Breakfast Recipes:

<u>Tuna Noodle Casserole</u>

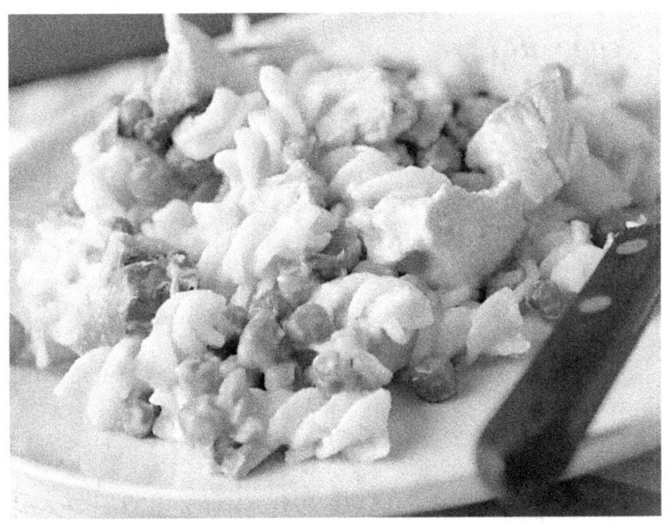

Ingredients:

- 8 ounce elbow macaroni noodles
- One (10.5 oz) can of condensed cream of mushroom soup
- 1/2 cup milk

- Drained and flaked one (5 oz) can of tuna in water
- 1 cup frozen peas
- 1/2 cup shredded cheddar cheese
- 1/4 cup chopped onion

Preparation:

1. Preheat your oven to 375°F (190°C). Cook macaroni noodles according to package guidelines. Drain and set aside.
2. Whisk together soup, milk, tuna, peas, and onion in a bowl.
3. Stir in cooked noodles and spoon mixture into a greased baking dish.
4. Top with shredded cheese.
5. Allow to bake for 20-25 minutes or until bubbling and golden brown. And enjoy

Nutritional Value (per serving):

- Calories: 300, Protein: 20g,

- Fat: 10g, Carbs: 30g

Cooking Time: 45 minutes

Servings: 4

frittata with Cottage Cheese and Vegetables

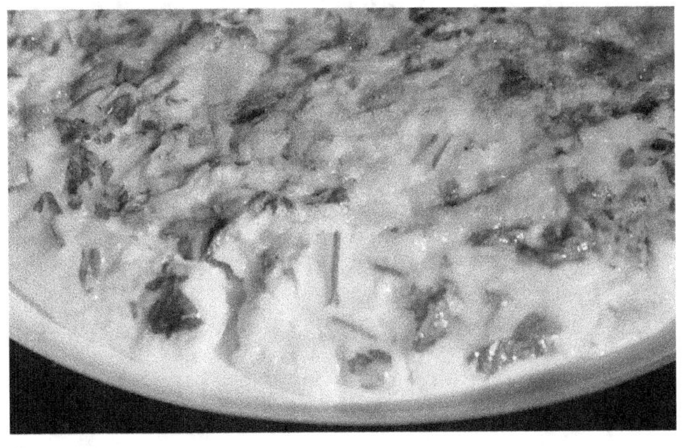

Ingredients:

Base:

- 2 large eggs (or 1/2 cup broken tofu for egg substitute)

- 1/4 cup plain plant-based milk (or milk of choice)
- 1/4 cup shredded low-fat mozzarella cheese (optional)
- Salt and pepper to taste

Filling:

- 1 tablespoon olive oil
- 1/2 cup chopped onion
- 1/2 cup chopped bell pepper (any color)
- 1/4 cup chopped mushrooms
- 1/4 cup chopped spinach
- 1/4 cup broken cooked sausage (optional) - Skip for vegetarian choice
- 1/4 cup crumbled cottage cheese

Preparation:

1. Preheat your oven to 375°F (190°C). Grease a small oven-safe pan or pie dish.

2. Whisk together the eggs (or broken tofu), milk, cheese (if using), salt, and pepper in a bowl. Set aside.

3. Heat your olive oil in the pan over medium heat and add onion, bell pepper, and mushrooms. Cook until melted, about 5 minutes.

4. Stir in chopped spinach and cook for another minute, or until wilted.

5. Optional: If using cooked meat, add it to the pan and cook for another minute.

6. Pour the egg or tofu mixture over the veggies in the skillet.

7. Sprinkle the broken cottage cheese on top.

8. Bake in the prepared oven for 20-25 minutes, or until the frittata is set and golden brown on top.

9. Serve: Cut into wedges and eat warm.

Nutritional Value (per dish - with eggs and sausage):

- Calories: 400

- Protein: 30g

- Fat: 20g

- Carbohydrates: 20g (Egg Substitute Option):

Cooking Time: 30 minutes

Serving: 2

- *Replace eggs with crumbled tofu for a vegan choice. Season the tofu with a pinch of turmeric for a more "eggy" taste.*

Omelet with Vegetables

Ingredients:

Omelet:

- 1/4 cup chickpea flour

- 1/4 cup water

- 1/4 teaspoon turmeric powder

- Salt and pepper to taste

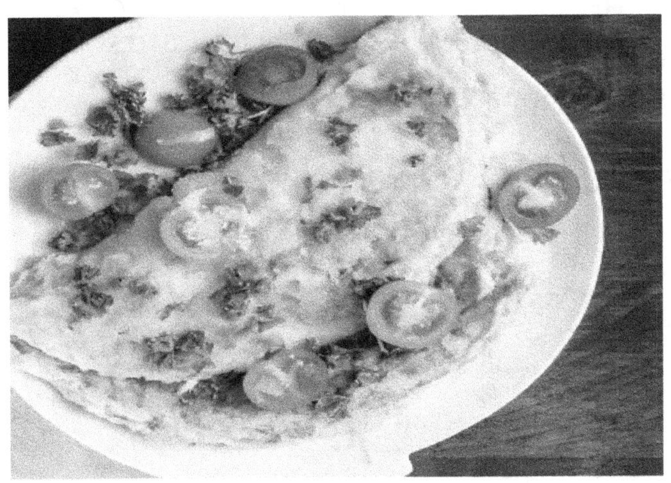

Filling:

- 1 tablespoon olive oil

- 1/4 cup chopped onion

- 1/4 cup chopped bell pepper (any color)

- 1/4 cup chopped mushrooms

- 1/4 cup crumbled feta cheese (optional)

- 1 tablespoon chopped fresh parsley

Preparation:

1. In a small bowl, mix chickpea flour, water, turmeric powder, salt, and pepper. Allow the batter to rest for 5 minutes.

2. Heat your olive oil in a nonstick pan over medium heat. Then add onion and cook until softened, about 3 minutes.

3. Stir in chopped bell pepper and mushrooms. Then cook for an extra 2 minutes.

4. Pour the chickpea flour batter into the pan, swirling to coat the bottom. leave it to cook for 2-3 minutes, or until the bottom is set.

5. Optional: Sprinkle chopped feta cheese over one-half of the omelet.

6. Fold the other half over the center. Allow to cook for an extra 1-2 minutes, or until cooked through.

7. *Serve:* Plate the omelet and top with chopped fresh parsley. Enjoy!

Nutritional Value (per serve - with cheese):

- Calories: 350

- Protein: 20g

- Fat: 15g

Cooking Time: 20 minutes

Serving: 1

Breakfast Quesadillas with Black Beans and Scrambled Eggs

Ingredients:

Quesadilla:

- 1 whole wheat tortilla

- 1/4 cup shredded low-fat cheese (such as cheddar or Monterey Jack)

- 1/4 cup cooked black beans, cleaned and drained
- 1 large scrambled egg (or 1/4 cup broken tofu)
- Pinch of chili sauce (optional)
- Chopped fresh cilantro (optional)

Preparation:

1. Heat a lightly oiled pan over medium heat.

2. Place the tortilla on the pan. Sprinkle half with cheese, black beans, and scrambled egg (or broken tofu).

3. If using, sprinkle with a pinch of chili sauce.

4. Fold the tortilla in half, pressing down gently. Allow to cook for 2-3 minutes per side, or until golden brown and the cheese is melted.

5. ***Serve:*** Cut the quesadilla into wedges and top with chopped fresh cilantro (optional).

Nutritional Value (per serve - with egg):

- Calories: 350

- Protein: 20g

- Fat: 15g

- Carbohydrates: 30g

Cooking Time: 15 minutes

Serving: 1

Spicy Sausage and Egg Scramble with Sweet Potato Hash

Ingredients:

Scrambled Eggs:

- 2 big eggs

- 1/4 cup plain plant-based milk (or milk of choice)

- 1/4 teaspoon smoked pepper

- Pinch of chili pepper (optional)
- Salt and pepper to taste

Spicy Sausage (optional):

- 2 ounces cooked and broken breakfast sausage

Sweet Potato Hash:

- 1 tablespoon olive oil
- 1 medium sweet potato, diced
- 1/2 cup chopped bell pepper (any color)
- 1/4 cup chopped onion
- 1/4 teaspoon dried cumin
- Salt and pepper to taste

Preparation:

1. Preheat your oven to 400°F (200°C). Toss chopped sweet potato with a tablespoon of olive oil and spread on a baking sheet. Allow to roast for 15-20 minutes, or until tender-crisp.

2. While the sweet potato roasts, heat another tablespoon of olive oil in a pan over medium heat. Put onion and bell pepper. Then cook for 5 minutes, or until softened.

3. Optional: If using, add cooked and crumbled breakfast sausage to the pan and cook for an additional minute.

4. In a different bowl, whisk together eggs, milk, smoked paprika, cayenne pepper (optional), salt, and pepper.

5. Pour the egg mixture into the skillet with the veggies (and sausage, if using). Cook, stirring occasionally, until the eggs are mixed and cooked through.

6. *Serve:* Plate the scrambled eggs with the roasted sweet potato dish. Enjoy!

Nutritional Value (per serve - with cheese):

- Calories: 350

- Protein: 30-35g

- Fat: 15g

Cooking Time:30 minutes,

Serving: 2

Turkey and Veggie Frittata Muffins

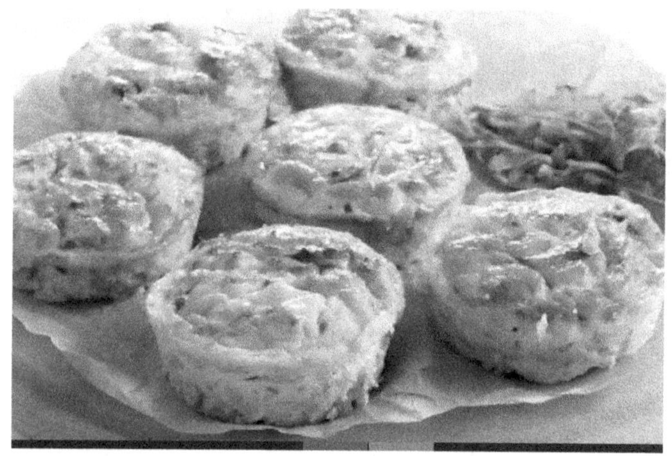

Ingredients:

Base:

- 8 big eggs

- 1/4 cup shredded low-fat cheese (such as cheddar or Monterey Jack)

- 1/4 cup plain plant-based milk (or milk of choice)
- 1/4 teaspoon dried oregano
- Salt and pepper to taste

Filling:

- 1 tablespoon olive oil
- 1/2 cup chopped onion
- 1/2 cup chopped bell pepper (any color)
- 1/2 cup chopped mushrooms
- 1/2 cup cooked and chopped ground turkey
- 1/4 cup chopped spinach

Preparation:

1. Preheat your oven to 375°F (190°C). Grease a muffin pan.
2. In a big bowl, whisk together eggs, cheese, milk, oregano, salt, and pepper. Then heat your olive oil in a

pan over medium heat. Add onion, bell pepper, and mushrooms and cook for 5 minutes, or until softened.

3. Stir in the cooked ground turkey and chopped spinach. Cook for an extra minute.

4. Divide the egg mixture equally among the greased muffin cups. Spoon the veggie and turkey mixture on top of each.

5. Bake for 20-25 minutes, or until the frittatas are set and golden brown on top.

6. *Serve:* Let the frittatas cool slightly before taking them from the muffin tin. Enjoy warm or at room temperature.

Nutritional value:

- Calories: 200

- Protein 20g
- Fat: 15

Cooking Time: 45 minutes

Serving: 6

Baked Chicken with Sweet Potato Mash

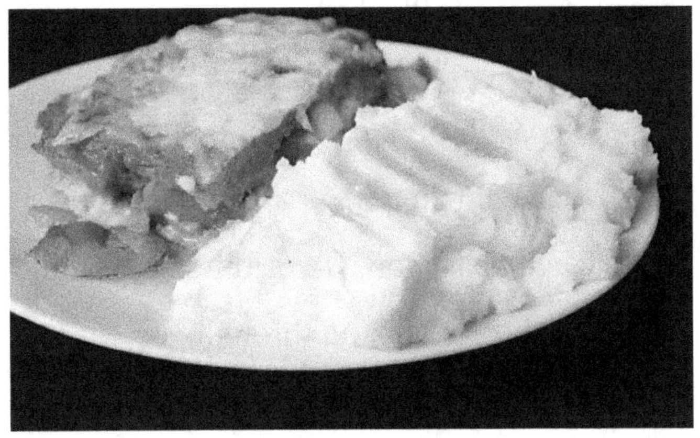

Ingredients:

- Two boneless, skinless chicken breasts
- 1 tablespoon olive oil
- 1/2 teaspoon dried thyme

- 1/4 teaspoon salt

- 1/4 teaspoon black pepper

- 1 medium sweet potato, peeled and chopped

- 1/4 cup milk

- 1 tablespoon butter, softened

Preparation:

1. Preheat your oven to 400°F (200°C).

2. In a bowl, mix chicken breasts with olive oil, thyme, salt, and pepper.

3. Place chicken in a baking dish.

4. Then roast for 20-25 minutes, or until chicken is cooked through.

5. While the chicken cooks, boil sweet potato until tender, about 15 minutes.

6. Drain the sweet potato and mash with milk and butter.

7. Serve chicken breasts with sweet potato mash.

Nutritional Value (per serving):

- Calories: 400

- Protein: 30g

- Fat: 15g, Carbs: 40g

Cooking Time: 45 minutes

Servings: 2

Coconut Blueberry Baked Oats

Ingredients:

- 2 cups rolled oats

- Half a cup (firmly packed) of shredded coconut

- 1 tsp ground cinnamon

- 1 tsp chopped ginger

- 1 tsp baking powder

- 1/4 tsp salt

- 3/4 cup walnuts

- One and a half cups of fresh or frozen blueberries

- 3 eggs
- Milk of your choice 440ml (about One and 3/4 cups)
- 3 tablespoons honey, brown rice syrup, or maple syrup
- 1 tbsp vanilla flavor
- Two tbsp melted butter or coconut oil

Preparation:

1. Preheat your oven to 180 C. Roughly break up the walnuts into halves and spread out on a small tray. Allow to toast for about 6 minutes or until lightly golden, then set aside to cool.

2. Combine oats, coconut, cinnamon, ginger, baking powder, and salt in a big bowl.

3. In a different bowl, whisk together the eggs, milk, honey (or other liquid

sweetener), vanilla, and melted butter/coconut oil.

4. Take a baking dish (I used a 24.5cm square baking dish) and lightly grease the sides with a dash of butter or oil. Scatter in half of the oat mixture and spread evenly across the base. Then layer in about a cup of the blueberries, followed by the rest of the oat mixture, walnuts, and finally the leftover blueberries.

5. Carefully pour the liquid mixture over the dish, making sure it spreads evenly and settles into the dry ingredients. Then try shaking the dish gently to help the liquid sink in.

6. Bake the mixture for approximately 45 minutes, or until the middle of the

bake feels firm and the top is a deep golden brown and slightly crispy.

7. To slice and store: allow the bake to cool to room temperature (it will set and slice easier if you allow it to cool first), then cut into pieces and store in a sealed container in the fridge. It can last up to five days if stored in the fridge.

Nutritional Value per serving:

- Protein 9.1g
- Carbs 30.8g
- Fiber 3.7g

Serving: 2-3

Cooking Time: 50 minutes

Berry Banana Crumble Muesli Bars

Ingredients:

WET INGREDIENTS:

- 1 egg
- 1/3 cup honey or maple syrup
- 100mL extra virgin olive oil or butter

DRY INGREDIENTS:

- 3/4 cup (110g) of different seeds such as linseeds, sunflower seeds, and sesame
- One cup of gluten-free (160g) or wholemeal plain flour
- One cup (86g) quinoa flakes
- One cup (52g) chopped coconut
- Half cup (52g) dried coconut
- One tbsp ground cinnamon

FILLING:

- One cup of berries, fresh or frozen and defrosted
- One banana, sliced
- One tbsp vanilla flavor

Preparation:

1. Preheat your oven to 180C and line a big baking dish (20cm x 20cm) with greaseproof paper.

2. In a mixing bowl add all wet ingredients and whisk well.

3. In another big bowl combine all dry ingredients, mix, then add wet ingredients to dry ingredients and mix again.

4. Pour half the mix into the baking dish, press out equally using your hands then place in the oven to cook for 10 minutes.

5. While cooking, mix together ingredients for filling.

6. Once the base is cooked, pour in the filling and then top with the rest of the muesli mix. You can move around a

little so some berries poke through if you wish, then place in the oven and allow to cook for a further 30 minutes.

7. Allow to cool fully in tin, before slicing and serving.

8. It can last only for 5 days if stored in the fridge

- ***Note:*** *For a gluten-free alternative, use plain flour instead of wholemeal flour*

- *For a dairy-free alternative, use extra virgin olive oil instead of butter*

Nutritional Value per serving:

- Protein 3.6g

- Fat 11.4g, Carbs 15.7g

- Fiber 3.4g

Serving: 2-3

Cooking Time: 50 minutes

Banana & Chocolate Smoothie

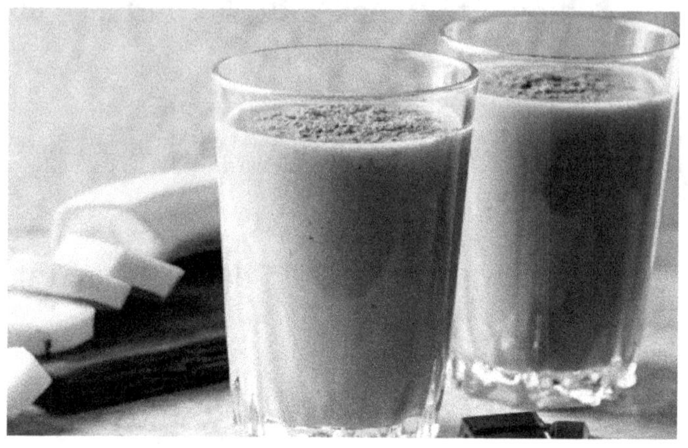

Ingredients:

- 1 ripe banana, frozen (easier to mix)
- 1/2 cup plain Greek yogurt (protein source)
- 1/2 cup milk (dairy or plant-based)
- 1 tablespoon unsweetened cocoa powder
- 1/4 cup chopped spinach (optional, for extra benefits)

- Ice cubes (optional, for thicker consistency)
- One Tbsp. of maple syrup or honey (optional, for sweetness)

Preparation:

1. In your blender add all your ingredients and blend until smooth and creamy.
2. serve in a glass and enjoy

Nutritional Value (approximate):

- Calories: 250, Protein: 15g
- Carbs: 35g, Fat: 5g

Preparation Time: 2 minutes

Serving: 1

Fried Eggs with Spiced Avocado

Ingredients:

- 2 big eggs
- 1/2 ripe avocado, mashed

- 1/4 teaspoon chili spice

- 1/8 teaspoon cumin

- Salt and pepper to taste

- 1 tablespoon olive oil

- 1 slice whole-wheat toast (optional)

Preparation:

1. Mash the avocado in a bowl and season with chili powder, cumin, salt, and pepper.

2. Warm up your olive oil in a pan over medium heat.

3. Crack the eggs into the pan and fry them to your chosen doneness.

4. Spread the avocado mash on the toast (if using).

5. Place the fried eggs on top of the avocado toast or serve them alongside.

Nutritional Value (approximate):

- Calories: 350

- Protein: 12g (from eggs)

- Carbs: 15g (from toast, if used)

- Fat: 20g (from avocado, olive oil)

Cooking Time: 5 minutes

Serving: 1

Scrambled Eggs with Smoked Salmon and Cottage Cheese

Ingredients:

- 2 big eggs

- 2 tablespoons crushed smoked salmon

- 1/4 cup low-fat cottage cheese

- 1/4 cup chopped fresh chives

- Salt and pepper to taste

- 1 tablespoon olive oil

Preparation:

1. Whisk the eggs in a bowl with a splash of water or milk. Season with

salt and pepper and heat your olive oil in a pan over medium heat.

2. Pour in the egg mixture and beat gently until cooked through.

3. Fold in the smoked salmon and cottage cheese, letting them warm slightly.

4. Garnish with fresh chives before serving.

Nutritional Value (approximate):

- Calories: 300

- Protein: 20g (from eggs, salmon, cottage cheese). Carbs: 5g

- Fat: 15g (from olive oil, fish)

Cooking Time: 5 minutes

Serving: 1

Cottage Cheese Pancakes with Berries and Nuts

Ingredients:

- 1/2 cup low-fat cottage cheese
- 1/4 cup whole-wheat flour
- 1 egg
- 1/4 teaspoon baking powder
- Pinch of salt
- 1/4 cup milk (dairy or plant-based)
- 1/4 cup mixed berries
- 1 tablespoon crushed walnuts
- Maple syrup (extra, for topping)

Preparation:

1. In a bowl, mash the cottage cheese until smooth.
2. Whisk in the flour, egg, baking powder, and salt until a batter forms.
3. Warm your lightly oiled pan over medium heat.

4. Pour in 1/4 cup of batter per pancake and cook for 2-3 minutes per side or until golden brown.

5. While the pancakes cook, heat the berries in a small pot until slightly softened (optional).

6. Serve the pancakes topped with berries, walnuts, and a drizzle of maple syrup (optional).

Nutritional Value (approximate):

- Calories: 400

- Protein: 20g (from cottage cheese, egg) , Carbs: 40g

- Fat: 10g (from cottage cheese, peanuts)

Cooking Time: 10 minutes

Serving: 1

Mushroom-baked eggs with squashed tomatoes

Ingredients:

- Two big flat mushrooms (about 85g each), stalks removed, and chopped
- Rapeseed oil, for brushing
- Half garlic clove, grated (optional)
- a few thyme leaves
- Two tomatoes, split
- 2 big eggs
- 2 handfuls rocket

Preparation:

1. Warm your oven to 200C/180C.
2. Brush the mushrooms with a little oil and the garlic (if using). Then put your mushrooms in two very lightly greased gratin dishes, bottom-side up, and season lightly with pepper and top with the chopped stalks and

thyme, cover with foil, and bake for 20 mins.

3. Take out the foil, add the tomatoes to the dishes, and break an egg carefully onto each of the mushrooms. Season and add a little more thyme, if you like. Return to the oven for 10-12 mins or until the eggs are set but the whites are still runny.

4. Top with the lettuce and eat straight from the dishes.

Nutritional Value:

- Calories:147
- Carbs:5g
- fiber : 3g
- Protein :12g

Cooks Time: 30m/ Prep: 5m

Serving: 2

Breakfast burrito

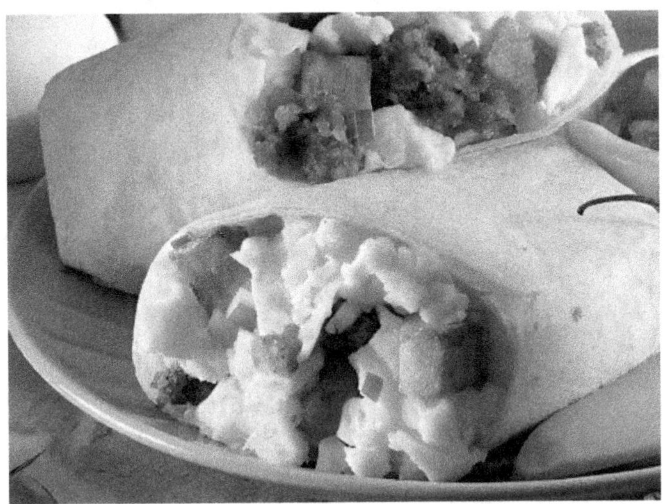

Ingredients:

- 1 tsp chipotle sauce

- 1 egg

- 1 tsp rapeseed oil 50g kale

- Seven cherry tomatoes halved

- Half a small avocado, sliced

- 1 wholemeal tortilla wrap, warmed

Preparation:

1. Whisk the chipotle paste with the egg
   and some salt in a jug. Heat the oil in

a big frying pan, add the kale and tomatoes.

2. Cook until the kale is limp and the tomatoes have softened, then push everything to the side of the pan. Pour the beaten egg into the cleaned half of the pan and scramble. Layer everything into the middle of your wrap, topping with the avocado, then wrap up and eat immediately.

Nutritional value per wrap:

- Calories 366, Carbs 26g
- fiber 5g
- protein 16g

Cooking Time: 15m

serve:1

Greek Yogurt Parfait with Berries and Granola

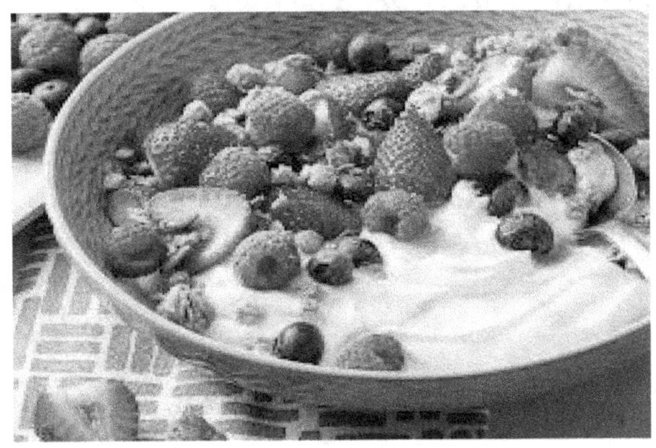

Ingredients:

- 1 cup plain Greek yogurt
- 1/2 cup mixed berries (fresh or frozen)
- 1/4 cup granola
- 1 tablespoon honey (optional)

Preparation:

1. Lay your Greek yogurt, berries, and granola in a glass or bowl.

2. Drizzle with honey (optional) for added sweetness and enjoy

Nutritional Value (per serving):

- Calories: 300
- Protein: 20g, Fat: 10g, Carbs: 30g

Cooking Time: 20 minutes

Servings: 1

Lunch Recipes:

Chicken & chorizo jambalaya

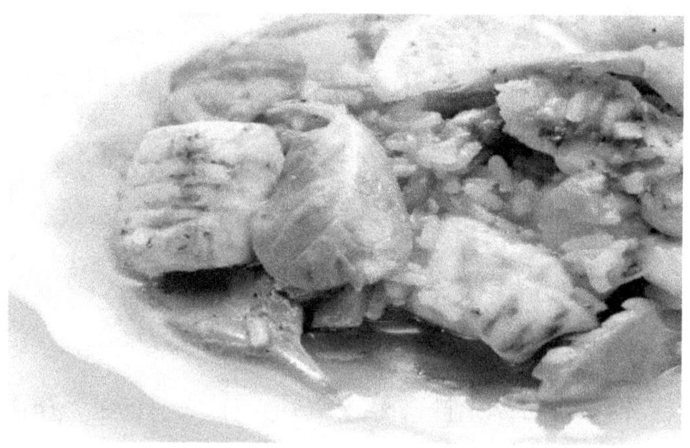

Ingredients:

- A tablespoon of olive oil

- 2 chicken breasts, sliced
- 1 onion, diced
- 1 red pepper, neatly sliced
- Two garlic cloves, crushed
- 75g chorizo, sliced
- 1 tbsp Cajun seasoning
- 250g long grain rice
- 400g of plum tomato
- 350ml chicken stock

Preparation:

1. Heat olive oil in a large frying pan with a cover and cook chopped chicken breasts for 5-8 mins until browned. Remove and set aside.

2. Tip in the diced onion and simmer for 3-4 mins until tender.

3. Add thinly sliced red pepper, crushed garlic cloves, sliced chorizo, and Cajun seasoning, and simmer for 5

mins more then stir the chicken back in with long grain rice, add the tomatoes, and chicken stock. Cover and boil for 20-25 mins until the rice is cooked. Allow to cool and serve

Nutritional value per serving:

- Calories:445, Carbs:64g
- Protein:30g, Fiber:2g, Fat: 10

Cooking Tim3: 45 min/prep:10 min

Serve: 4

Salade niçoise (Classic French Dish)

Niçoise with Seared Tuna Steaks

Ingredients:

- 2 tuna steaks (each about 6 oz)
- 1 tablespoon olive oil
- Salt and freshly ground black pepper
- 4 tiny red potatoes, halved and cooked

- 1 cup green beans, trimmed and blanched
- 1/2 cup cherry tomatoes, halved
- 1 head of romaine lettuce, chopped
- 1/2 cup pitted Kalamata olives
- 2 hard-boiled eggs, quartered
- 2 tablespoons Dijon mustard
- 2 teaspoons red wine vinegar
- 1 tablespoon olive oil
- 1 tablespoon fresh lemon juice
- Freshly cut parsley, for garnish (optional)

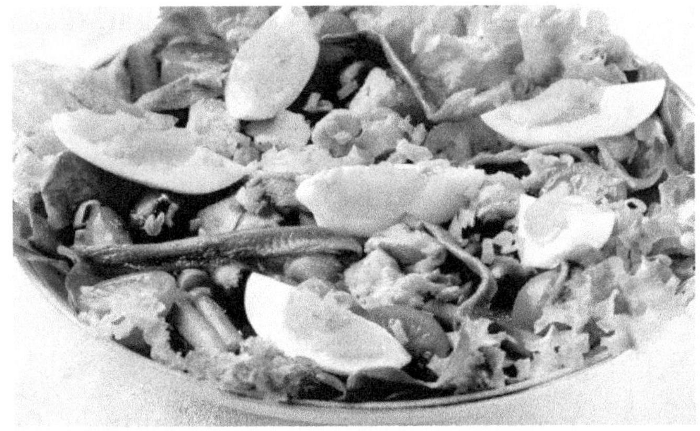

Preparation:

1. Pat tuna steaks dry and add salt and pepper. Then heat your olive oil in a large skillet over medium-high heat. Sear tuna steaks for 2-3 minutes per side for a rare sear, or longer for preferred doneness.

2. While tuna sears, make the salad. In a large bowl, add cooked potatoes, green beans, cherry tomatoes, and chopped romaine lettuce.

3. In a separate bowl, whisk together Dijon mustard, red wine vinegar, olive oil, and lemon juice for the dressing.

4. *To assemble the salad:* Arrange salad ingredients on a plate. Top with seared tuna steaks, Kalamata olives, and quartered hard-boiled eggs. Drizzle with dressing and top with

fresh parsley (optional) before serving.

Nutritional Value (per serving):

- Calories: 500
- Protein: 40g
- Fat: 25g
- Carbs: 30g

Cooking Time: 30 minutes

Serving: 2

Niçoise with Chickpeas and Grilled Chicken

Ingredients:

- 1 boneless, skinless chicken breast
- 1 tablespoon olive oil
- Salt and freshly ground black pepper
- One can (15 oz) of chickpeas, rinsed and drained

- 4 small red potatoes, halved and cooked
- 1 cup green beans, trimmed and blanched
- 1/2 cup cherry tomatoes, halved
- 1 head of romaine lettuce, chopped
- 1/2 cup pitted Kalamata olives
- 2 hard-boiled eggs, quartered
- 2 teaspoons red wine vinegar
- 1 tablespoon olive oil
- 1 tablespoon fresh lemon juice
- One tablespoon chopped fresh herbs (basil, oregano, or parsley)
- Freshly cut parsley, for garnish (optional)

Preparation:

1. Marinate chicken breast in olive oil, salt, and pepper for at least 30 minutes. Preheat your grill to

medium-high heat. Grill the chicken breast for 10-15 minutes per side, or until cooked through.

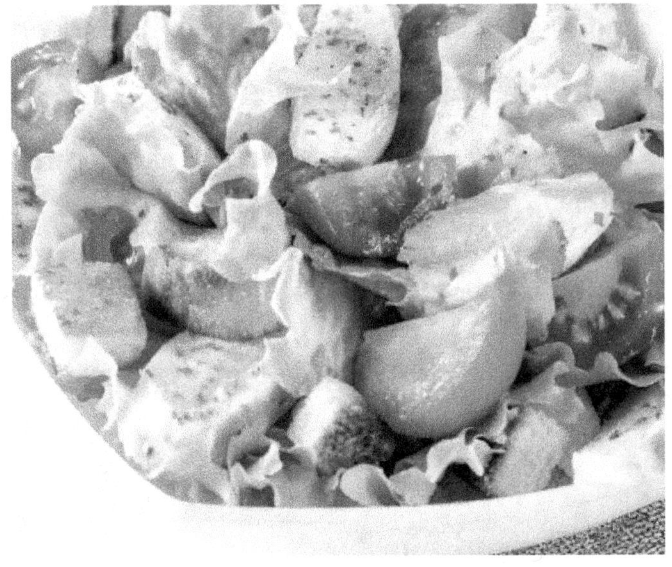

2. While the chicken grills, prepare the salad. In a large bowl, add cooked potatoes, green beans, cherry tomatoes, and chopped romaine lettuce.

3. In a separate bowl, whisk together red wine vinegar, olive oil, lemon juice,

and chopped fresh herbs for the dressing.

4. ***To assemble the salad:*** Arrange salad ingredients on a plate. Top with sliced grilled chicken, chickpeas, Kalamata olives, and quartered hard-boiled eggs. Drizzle with dressing and top with fresh parsley (optional) before serving.

Nutritional Value (per serving):

- Calories: 400
- Protein: 30g
- Fat: 20g
- Carbs: 20g

Cooking Time: 45 minutes (including grilling time)

Serving: 2

- *This variation includes chickpeas and grilled chicken for a vegetarian protein option.*

Niçoise with Smoked Salmon and Poached Eggs

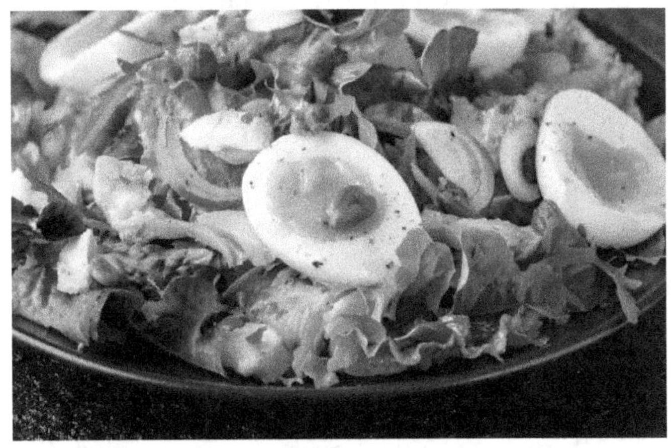

Ingredients:

- 4 slices smoked salmon
- 4 eggs
- 1 tablespoon white vinegar
- 4 small red potatoes, halved and cooked

- 1 cup green beans, trimmed and blanched
- 1/2 cup cherry tomatoes, halved
- 1 head of romaine lettuce, chopped
- 1/2 cup pitted Kalamata olives
- 2 teaspoons Dijon mustard
- 2 teaspoons red wine vinegar
- 1 tablespoon olive oil
- Freshly chopped chives, for garnish (optional)

Preparation:

1. ***Poach eggs:*** Bring a pot of water to a simmer. Add vinegar. Crack each egg into a small bowl. Gently swirl the water and carefully spoon each egg into the heating water. Cook for 3-4 minutes, or until whites are set and yolks are runny.

2. While eggs poach, prepare the salad. In a large bowl, add cooked potatoes, green beans, cherry tomatoes, and chopped romaine lettuce.

3. In a separate bowl, whisk together Dijon mustard, red wine vinegar, olive oil, and fresh herbs (optional) for the dressing.

4. ***To assemble the salad:*** present the salad on a plate. Top with smoked salmon slices, poached eggs, and Kalamata olives. Drizzle with dressing and top with fresh chives (optional) before serving.

Nutritional Value (per serving):

- Calories: 400
- Protein: 30g
- Fat: 20g
- Carbs: 20g

Serving: 2

Spiced chicken kebabs with chopped salad & flatbreads

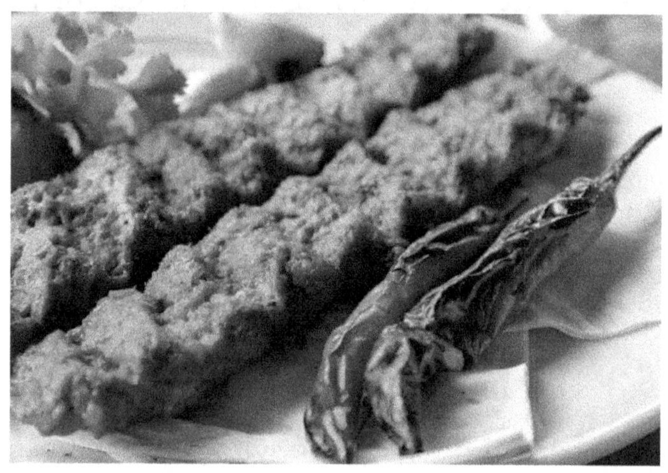

Ingredients:

- 200g Greek yogurt
- ½ tsp ground cinnamon (optional)
- 2 green cardamom pods, pods bashed and seeds finely crushed (optional)
- 1 tsp ground cumin

- 1 tsp ground turmeric

- pinch of chili flakes, or to taste

- 2 garlic cloves, smashed

- 1 lemon, zested and halved

- 640g pack of diced chicken thighs

- 1 cucumber, peeled half coarsely grated and half finely chopped

- 1 Little Gem lettuce, thinly sliced

- 4 flatbreads hot sauce, to serve (optional)

Preparation:

1. Combine the 100g of yogurt with the 1 mashed garlic, lemon zest, and salt in a bowl. Tip in the chicken and swirl well to coat. Cover and leave to marinate in the fridge for at least 30 minutes or overnight.

2. Mix the grated cucumber and the remaining garlic into the remaining

yogurt, then season with a pinch each of salt and pepper. Set away in the fridge.

3. Mix the finely sliced cucumber and lettuce, then squeeze over one of the lemon halves and season with a good amount of salt. Cut the remaining lemon half into quarters. Heat the grill to a high or a big griddle pan over high heat.

4. Thread the marinated chicken pieces onto metal skewers, set on a tray, and cook on a hot grill or in the griddle pan for 10-12 mins, rotating periodically to ensure it cooks evenly and is scorched in areas. Then warm your flatbreads under the grill or in a toaster and serve the chicken in the flatbreads with the chopped salad and

cucumber yogurt. Pour slowly with hot sauce before serving, if you want.

Nutritional value per serving:

- Calories: 516
- fat: 20g, Carbs:42g
- fiber: 5g
- Protein: 41g

Cooking time: 45 minutes

Serving: 4

Spinach, sweet potato & lentil dhal

Ingredients:

- 1 tbsp sesame oil
- 1 red onion, finely chopped
- 1 garlic clove, crushed
- thumb-sized piece ginger, peeled and finely chopped
- 1 red chili, coarsely chopped
- 1½ tsp ground turmeric

- 1½ tsp ground cumin

- 2 sweet potatoes (approximately 400g/14oz), sliced into even slices

- 250g red split lentils

- 600ml vegetable stock

- 80g bag of spinach

- 4 spring onions, cut on the diagonal, to serve

- Half a small pack of Thai basil leaves torn, to serve

Preparation:

1. Firstly heat your sesame oil in a wide-based pan with a tight-fitting lid.

2. Add 1 finely chopped red onion and simmer over low heat for 10 mins, stirring periodically, until softened.

3. Add 1 crushed garlic clove, a finely chopped thumb-sized piece of ginger, and 1 finely chopped red chili,

simmer for 1 minute, then add 1½ tsp of turmeric and ground cumin and cook for 1 minute more.

4. Turn the heat to medium, add 2 sweet potatoes, cut into even chunks, and whisk everything together so the potato is coated in the spice mixture.

5. Tip in red split lentils, 600ml vegetable stock.

6. Bring the liquid to a boil, then reduce the heat, cover, and cook for 20 minutes until the lentils are soft and the potato is just holding its shape. Then taste and adjust the seasoning, and gently stir in the spinach. Once wilted, garnish with the 4 diagonally sliced spring onions and torn basil leaves to serve.

7. Alternatively, allow it to cool fully, then divide it between airtight containers and keep it in the fridge for a healthy lunchbox.

Nutritional value per serving:

- Calories:397, fat:5g
- Carbs:65g, fiber:11g
- Protein:18g

Cooking Time: 45 minutes

Serve:4

Chicken with crushed harissa chickpeas

Ingredients:

- Two tbsp rapeseed oil
- 1 onion, chopped
- 1 red pepper, thinly sliced
- 1 yellow pepper, thinly sliced
- 4 chicken breasts

- 1 tbsp za'atar

- 400g can chickpeas

- 1½ tbsp red harissa paste

- 150g baby spinach

- half a small bunch of parsley, and finely chopped

- lemon wedges, to serve

Preparation:

1. Warm 1 tbsp of oil in a frying pan over medium heat and cook the onions and peppers for 7 mins until softened and brown.

2. Meanwhile, lay the chicken between two sheets of baking parchment and lightly bash till about 2cm thick. Mix up the remaining oil and the za'atar, then rub over the chicken. Season to taste.

3. Heat your grill to high heat. Put the chicken on a baking pan lined with foil, and grill for 3-4 mins each side, or until brown and cooked through.

4. Then Heat the chickpeas in a skillet with the harissa paste and 2 tbsp water until warmed through, roughly mash with a potato masher.

5. Wilt the spinach in a pan with 1 tbsp of water or in the microwave in a heatproof bowl. Stir the pepper and onion combination, spinach, and parsley through the chickpeas.

6. Serve with the cut chicken and the lemon wedges for squeezing over.

Nutritional value per serving:

- Calories: 366, fat:12g
- Carbs:16g
- Fiber: 7g

- Protein:44g

Cooking Time: 15 minutes

Serve:4

<u>*Pasta salad*</u>

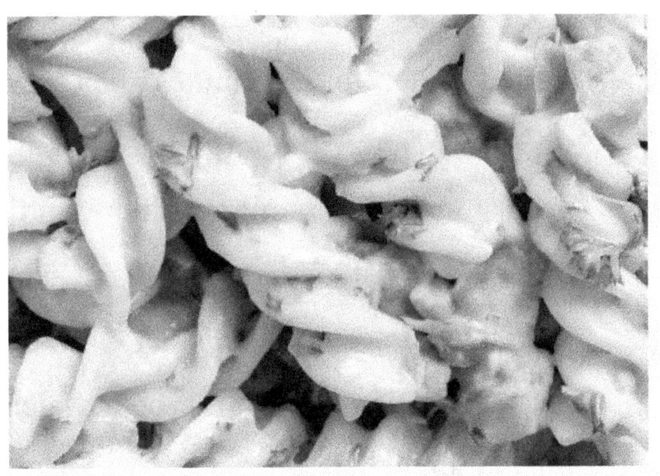

Ingredients:

- 300g farfalle (pasta bows)

- 200g frozen peas

- 1 big tomato fresh

- 10 sun dried tomatoes in oil

- 2 tbsp olive oil

- 2 tsp white wine vinegar
- 1 garlic clove
- huge fistful of fresh basil leaves
- 85g pack prosciutto or salami

Preparation:

1. ***COOK THE PASTA:*** Boil the pasta in salted water for 8 minutes then add the peas, return the water to a boil, and simmer for 2 minutes more until the pasta and peas are cooked. Tip into a colander over the sink, chill the pasta and peas under the cold water then drain well.

2. ***MAKE THE DRESSING:*** While the pasta is boiling, finely chop the tomato and put in a food processor with half the sun-dried tomatoes, the olive oil, vinegar, garlic, and around 8 basil leaves. Season salt and freshly

ground pepper then blitz till smooth. Tip into a large salad bowl.

3. ***TOSS AND SERVE:*** Add the pasta and peas to the vinaigrette, roughly slice the rest of the sun-dried tomatoes, and add to the pasta with the remaining basil leaves. Tear in the prosciutto or salami and toss everything together. Pile into bowls toast and enjoy.

Nutritional value per serving

- Calories: 426
- fat:12g carbs:64g fiber:6g
- protein:19g

Spicy Southwestern Black Bean Pasta Salad

Ingredients:

- 1 pound dry penne pasta, cooked according to package guidelines and cooled
- Washed and drained 1 (15-ounce) can of black beans
- 1 (10 oz) can corn, drained
- 1 red bell pepper, chopped
- 1 green bell pepper, chopped
- 1/2 red onion, thinly sliced
- 1 jalapeño pepper, seeded and finely chopped (optional, adjust for spice preference)
- 1/4 cup chopped fresh cilantro

Dressing:

- 1/4 cup olive oil
- 2 teaspoons lime juice
- 1 tablespoon red wine vinegar
- 1 teaspoon chili powder
- 1 teaspoon cumin

- 1/2 teaspoon smoked paprika

- Salt and freshly ground black pepper
  to taste

Preparation:

1. In a large bowl, add cooked pasta,
   black beans, corn, bell peppers, red
   onion, jalapeño (if using), and
   cilantro.

2. In a separate bowl, whisk together
   olive oil, lime juice, red wine vinegar,
   chili powder, cumin, smoked paprika,
   salt, and pepper.

3. Apply the dressing over the salad
   ingredients and toss to coat evenly.

4. Allow in the fridge for at least 30
   minutes before serving to enable the
   flavors to mingle.

Nutritional Value per serving:

- Calories: 400-450

- Protein: 20g (from black beans)

- Fat: 15-20g (from olive oil)

- Carbs: 50-55g (from pasta and corn)

Cooking Time: 30 minutes

Serves: 4-6

Greek Shrimp Pasta Salad with Feta and Spinach

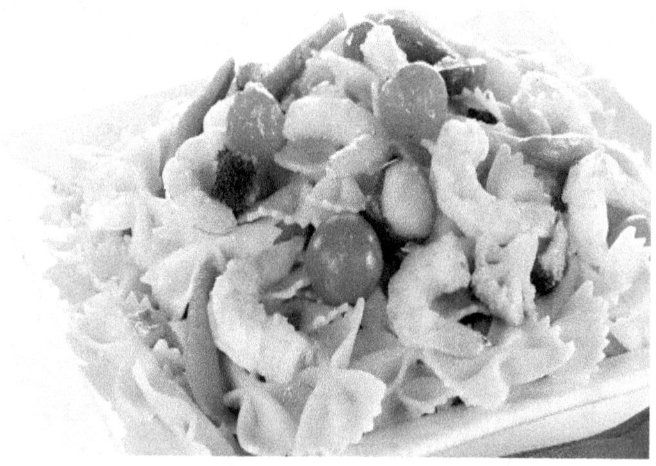

Ingredients:

- 1 pound dried farfalle pasta (bowtie), cooked according to package directions and cooled
- 1 pound cooked and deveined shrimp, cut into bite-sized pieces
- 1 cup crumbled feta cheese
- 1/2 cup chopped fresh spinach
- 1/4 cup chopped red onion
- 1/4 cup kalamata olives, pitted and halved

Dressing:
- 1/4 cup olive oil
- 2 teaspoons lemon juice
- 1 tablespoon red wine vinegar
- 1 teaspoon dried oregano
- 1/2 teaspoon garlic powder
- Salt and freshly ground black pepper to taste

Preparation:

1. In a large bowl, combine cooked pasta, shrimp, feta cheese, spinach, red onion, and kalamata olives.

2. In a separate bowl, whisk together olive oil, lemon juice, red wine vinegar, oregano, garlic powder, salt, and pepper to make a dressing.

3. Apply the dressing over the salad ingredients and toss to coat evenly.

4. Allow in the fridge for at least 30 minutes before serving to enable the flavors to mingle.

Nutritional Value per serving:

- Calories: 400-450
- Protein: 20g
- Fat: 20-25g
- Carbs: 40-45g

Cooking Time: 30 minutes

Serves: 4-6

Ingredients:

- 4 oz boneless, skinless chicken breast
- 1 cup cooked quinoa
- 2 cups mixed salad greens (spinach, arugula,)
- 1/2 cup cherry tomatoes, split
- 1/4 cup cucumber, sliced
- 1/4 cup feta cheese, crumbled
- 1 tablespoon olive oil
- 1 tablespoon balsamic vinegar
- Salt and pepper to taste

Preparation:

1. Season chicken breast with salt and pepper.
2. Grill the chicken until fully cooked (approximately 6-8 minutes per side).

3. In a big bowl, mix cooked quinoa, salad greens, cherry tomatoes, cucumber, and feta cheese.

4. Slice the cooked chicken and place it on top of the salad.

5. Drizzle with olive oil and balsamic vinegar.

6. Toss gently to mix.

Nutritional Value (Approx.):

- Protein: 30g
- Fiber: 6g, Calories: 400

Cooking Time: 20 minutes

Serving Size: 1

Lentil and Vegetable Soup

Ingredients:

- 1 cup dry green or brown lentil
- 1 onion, diced
- 2 carrots, peeled and chopped

- 2 celery stalks, chopped
- 2 cloves garlic, minced
- 4 cups low-sodium veggie broth
- 1 can (14 oz) diced tomatoes
- 1 teaspoon dried thyme
- Salt and pepper to taste

Preparation:

1. Rinse lentils thoroughly.
2. In a big pot, sauté onions, carrots, celery, and garlic until softened.
3. Add lentils, veggie broth, diced tomatoes, thyme, salt, and pepper.
4. Bring to a boil, then reduce heat and simmer for 25-30 minutes or until lentils are soft.
5. Adjust salt as needed.Serve and enjoy

Nutritional Value (Approx.):

- Protein: 18g, Fiber: 12g
- Calories: 350

Cooking Time: 40 minutes

Serving Size: 2 serves

Tofu and Vegetable Stir-Fry with Brown Rice

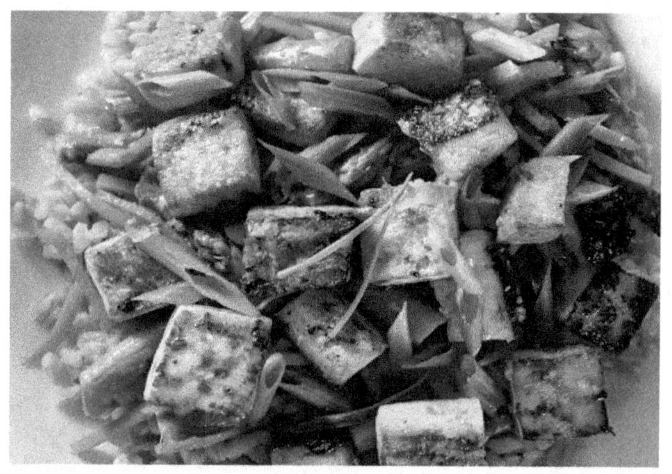

Ingredients:

- 8 oz firm tofu, cubed
- 1 cup broccoli stems
- 1 bell pepper, sliced
- 1 carrot, julienned
- 2 tablespoons soy sauce

- 1 tablespoon sesame oil

- 1 teaspoon ginger, grated

- 1 clove garlic, minced

- 1 cup cooked brown rice

Preparation:

1. Press tofu to remove extra water, then cut into cubes.

2. Heat sesame oil in a pan and add tofu, cooking until golden brown.

3. Add broccoli, bell pepper, carrot, ginger, and garlic. Stir-fry until the veggies are tender.

4. Pour soy sauce over the mixture and stir to combine.

5. Serve over cooked brown rice.

Nutritional Value (Approx.):

- Protein: 20g, Fiber: 6g

- Calories: 380

Cooking Time: 25 minutes

Baked Salmon with Quinoa and Roasted Vegetables

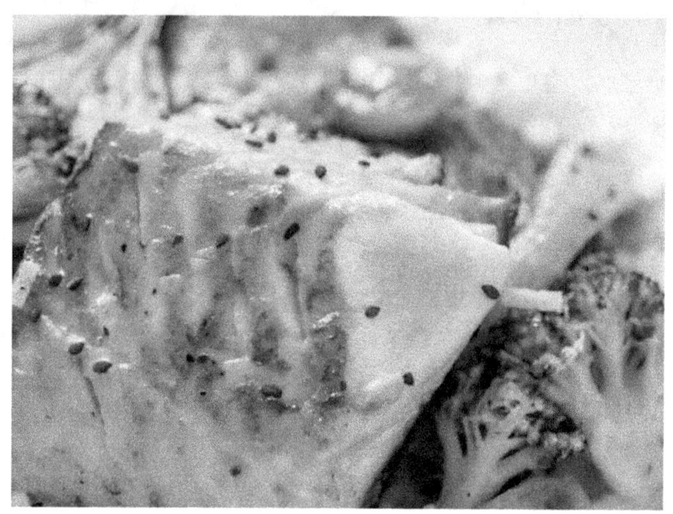

Ingredients:

- 6 oz salmon piece
- 1/2 cup quinoa, cooked
- 1 cup mixed veggies (e.g., bell peppers, zucchini, cherry tomatoes)
- 1 tablespoon olive oil

- 1 teaspoon dried herbs (rosemary, thyme, or your choice)
- Salt and pepper to taste
- Lemon wedges for serving

Preparation:

1. Preheat the oven to 400°F (200°C).

2. Place salmon on a baking sheet and surround it with mixed veggies.

3. Drizzle olive oil over salmon and veggies, and sprinkle with dried herbs, salt, and pepper.

4. Bake in the hot oven for 15-20 minutes or until the salmon is cooked through.

5. Serve the baked salmon over a bed of cooked rice, with lemon wedges on the side.

Nutritional Value (Approx.):

- Protein: 32g , Fiber: 6g

- Calories: 450

Cooking Time: 25 minutes

Serving Size: 1 serving

Dinner Recipes:

Spaghetti bolognese

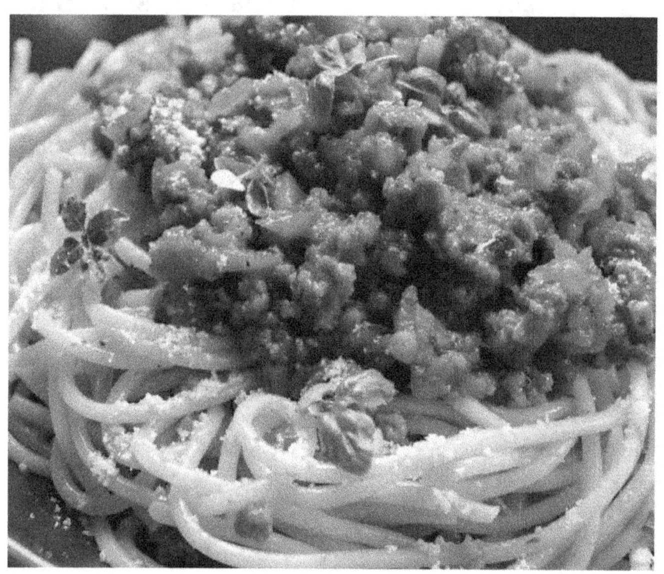

Ingredients:

- 1 tbsp olive oil

- 4 rashers smoked streaky bacon,
  finely chopped

- 2 medium onions, finely chopped

- 2 carrots, clipped and finely chopped

- 2 celery sticks, finely chopped

- 2 garlic cloves finely chopped

- Two or Three sprigs of rosemary leaves picked and finely chopped

- 500g meat mince

For the bolognese sauce:

- 2 x 400g tins plum tomatoes

- small pack of basil leaves picked, ¾ finely chopped and the rest left whole for garnish

- 1 tsp dried oregano

- 2 fresh bay leaves

- 2 tbsp tomato purée

- 1 beef stock cube

- 1 red chili deseeded and finely chopped (optional)

- 125ml red wine

- 6 cherry tomatoes sliced in half

To season and serve:

- 75g parmesan grated, plus extra to serve
- 400g spaghetti
- crusty bread to serve (optional)

Preparation:

1. Put a big saucepan on a medium heat and add 1 tbsp olive oil.

2. Put finely chopped bacon rashers and fry for 10 mins until golden and crisp.

3. Reduce the heat and add the onions, carrots, celery sticks, garlic cloves, and the leaves from sprigs rosemary, all finely chopped, then fry for 10 mins and stir the veg often until it softens.

4. Increase the heat to medium-high, add 500g beef mince, and cook stirring for

3-4 mins until the meat is browned all over.

5. Pour in plum tomatoes, finely chopped basil leaves, dried oregano, bay leaves, tomato purée, 1 beef stock cube, 1 deseeded and finely chopped red chili (if using), 125ml red wine, and 6 split cherry tomatoes and stir with a wooden spoon, breaking up the plum tomatoes.

6. Carry to a boil, reduce to a gentle simmer, and cover with a lid. Cook for 1 hr 15 mins turning occasionally, until you have a rich, thick sauce.

7. Add your grated parmesan, check the spices and stir.

8. When the bolognese is nearly finished, cook 400g spaghetti following the pack directions.

9. Drain the spaghetti and either stir into the bolognese sauce or serve the sauce on top. Serve with more grated parmesan, the leftover basil leaves, and crusty bread, if you like.

Nutritional value per serving:

- Calories: 624
- Fat:25g, Carbs: 58g
- fiber 6g
- Protein 35g

Cook: 1hr 50 min/Prep: 25

Serving: 6

Pork noodle stir-fry

Ingredients:

- 3 tbsp sesame oil
- 350g lean pork mince
- 350g egg noodles

- A thumb-sized piece of ginger peeled and chopped, or 1½ tbsp ginger purée

- Three garlic cloves, crushed, or 1 tbsp garlic purée

- 320g veggies (mangetout, baby sweetcorn, beansprouts, carrots, and peppers)

- 4 tbsp low-salt soy sauce

- 2 tsp cornflour

- 4 tbsp sweet chili sauce

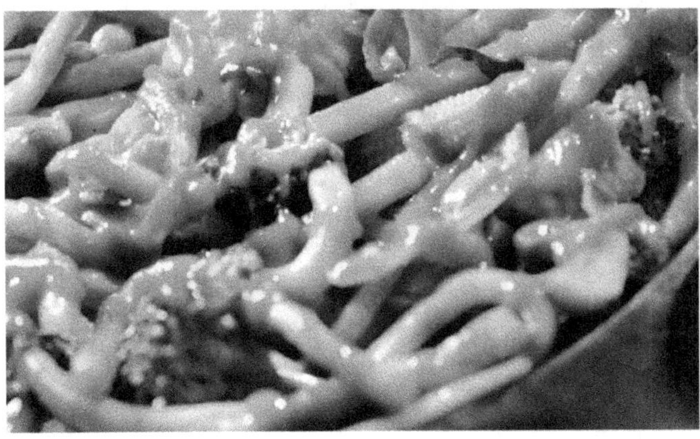

Preparation:

1. Heat your oil in a wok or cooking pan. Add the minced meat, break it up

104

with a spoon, and fry over high heat for about 8 minutes until browned. While the meat cooks, boil water, then pour the hot water over the noodles. Set aside for 5-10 mins to soften.

2. Put your ginger, garlic, and veggies in the pan and stir-fry for 2-3 mins. Mix one tablespoon of soy sauce with the cornflour to make a paste.

3. Add the leftover soy sauce, the chili sauce, and 2 tbsp water. After draining your noodles, put them in the pan with the sauce.

4. Allow to cook until the sauce coats the noodles, adding a splash of water if needed, then serve.

Nutritional Value per serving:
- Calories: 599, Fat:19g
- Carbs: 74g fiber: 5g

- Protein: 31g

Cooking Time: 15 minutes

Server: 4

<u>*Vegetable & bean chili*</u>

Ingredients:

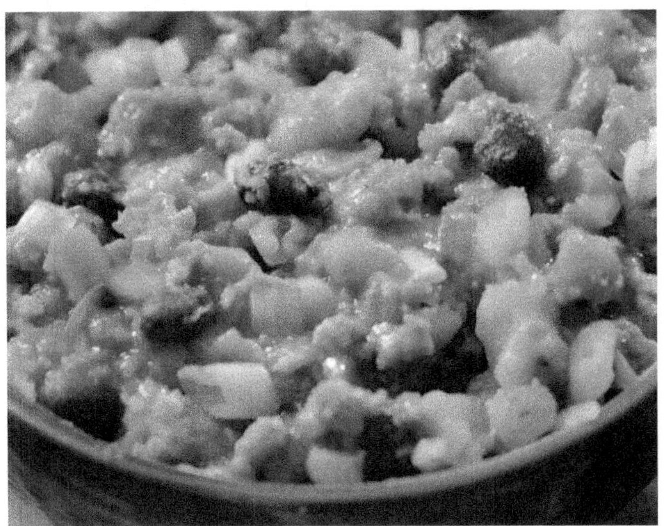

- 1 tbsp olive oil

- One clove garlic, finely chopped

- 1 ginger, finely chopped

- 1 big onion, chopped

- Two courgettes, diced

- 1 red pepper, deseeded and chopped
- 1 yellow pepper, deseeded and chopped
- 1 tbsp chili pepper
- 100g red lentils, washed and drained
- 1 tbsp tomato purée
- 2x cans chopped tomatoes
- 195g can sweetcorn, drained
- 420g can butter beans, drained
- 400g can kidney beans in water, drained

Preparation:

1. Heat the oil in a big pan and cook your garlic, ginger, onion, courgettes, and peppers for about 5 minutes until starting to soften. Put the chili powder and cook for 1 minute more.

2. Stir in the lentils, tomato purée, tomatoes, and 250ml water. Then

carry to a boil and cook for 15-20 mins.

3. Add the sweetcorn and beans, and cook for a further 10 minutes. Carry down, allow it to chill and enjoy.

Nutritional Value per serving:

- Calories: 361, Fat: 6g
- Carbs: 61g, Fiber: 13g
- Protein: 21g

Grilled Chicken with Rice & Vegetable Salad

Ingredients:

Chicken:

- 1 boneless, skinless chicken breast (4-5 oz)
- 1/2 tablespoon olive oil
- Salt and pepper to taste

Rice:

- 1/2 cup cooked brown rice (or any favorite cooked grain)

Salad:

- 1/2 cup mixed greens (chopped)
- 1/4 cup cherry tomatoes, halved
- 1/4 cup cucumber, sliced
- 1 tablespoon chopped feta cheese (optional)
- 1 tablespoon olive oil and vinegar sauce (or light vinaigrette of choice)

Preparation:

1. Warm your grill or grill pan to medium-high heat.
2. Apply olive oil, salt, and pepper to the chicken. Then grill chicken for 5-7 minutes per side, or until cooked through.

3. While your chicken cooks, make the salad by combining greens, tomatoes, and cucumber in a bowl.

4. Once cooked, slice the chicken and add it to the salad.

5. Drizzle with sauce and top with feta cheese (if using) before serving.

Nutritional Value (per serving):

- Calories: 400

- Protein: 30g

- Fat: 12g

- Carbohydrates: 35g

Cooking time: 45 minutes

Serving: 1

Honey Garlic Glazed Pork Chops with Sauteed Green Beans

Ingredients:

- 4 boneless pork chops (approximately 1-inch thick)
- 1 tablespoon olive oil
- 1/4 cup honey
- 2 teaspoons soy sauce
- 1 tablespoon Dijon mustard
- 1 tablespoon rice vinegar
- 1 clove garlic, minced
- 1 pound fresh green beans, trimmed and sliced into bite-sized pieces
- Salt and freshly ground black pepper to taste

Preparation:

1. In a small bowl, stir together honey, soy sauce, Dijon mustard, rice vinegar, and garlic.

2. Warm your olive oil in a large skillet over medium-high heat and season pork chops with salt and pepper. Sear

pork chops for 2-3 minutes per side, or until golden brown.

3. Pour the honey-soy sauce glaze into the skillet and heat to a simmer. Reduce heat and simmer for 5-7 minutes, or until the glaze thickens slightly, intermittently spooning the glaze over the pork chops.

4. While the pork chops simmer, heat a separate skillet with a little oil and cook green beans until tender-crisp, seasoned with salt and pepper.

5. Serve pork chops with the glaze and sautéed green beans.

Nutritional Information (per serving):
- Calories: 450
- Protein: 35g, Fat: 20g
- Carbohydrates: 30g

Cooking Time: 30 minutes

Dijon Pork Chops with Creamy Mushroom Sauce and Asparagus

Ingredients:

- 4 bone-in pork chops (approximately 1-inch thick)
- 2 tablespoons olive oil
- 1 tablespoon Dijon mustard
- 1/2 teaspoon dried thyme
- 1/4 teaspoon salt
- 1/4 teaspoon black pepper
- 1 pound button mushrooms, sliced
- 1 shallot, minced
- 1 clove garlic, minced
- 1/2 cup white wine (optional)
- 1 cup chicken broth
- 1/4 cup heavy cream
- 1 tablespoon chopped fresh parsley

- 1 pound asparagus, trimmed

Preparation:

1. Preheat your oven to 400°F (200°C).

2. In a small bowl, mix Dijon mustard, thyme, salt, and pepper. Apply the mixture onto both sides of the pork chops.

3. Warm your olive oil in a large oven-proof pan over medium-high heat and sear pork chops for 2-3 minutes per side or until golden brown.

4. Take the pork chops out from the skillet and put aside.

5. Put mushrooms, shallot, and garlic into the pan and simmer until softened, about 5 minutes.

6. Deglaze the pan with white wine (if used), scraping away any browned

pieces. Let the wine simmer for a minute or two to decrease somewhat.

7. Add chicken broth and bring to a simmer. Cook for 5 minutes, or until the sauce thickens slightly.

8. Stir in heavy cream and minced parsley. Return the pork chops to the pan and nestle the asparagus spears around the pork chops.

9. Transfer the pan to the preheated oven and bake for 15-20 minutes, or until the pork chops are cooked through and the asparagus is tender-crisp.

Nutritional Value per serving:

- Calories: 400-500

- Protein: 25-30g Fat: 15-25g

- carbohydrates: 30-45g

Cooking Time: 45 minutes

Serves: 4

Bulgur Wheat Salad with Poached Egg

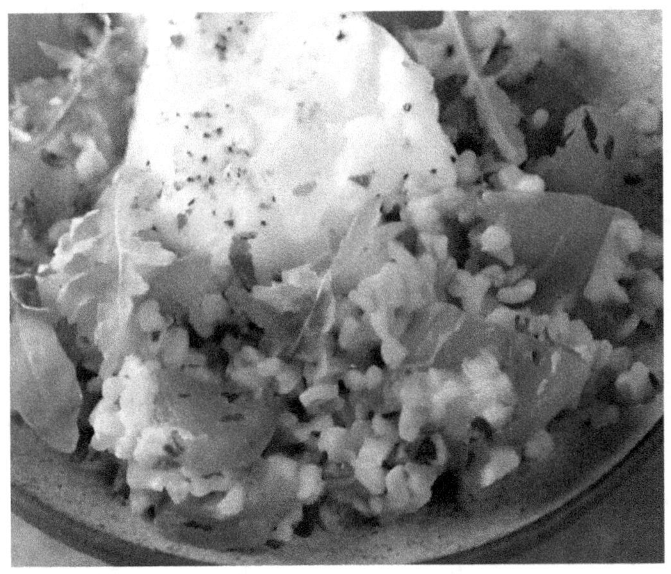

Ingredients:

- 1/2 cup cooked bulgur wheat
- 1/4 cup chopped cucumber
- 1/4 cup chopped tomato
- 1/4 cup chopped parsley
- 1 tablespoon chopped feta cheese (optional)

- 1 tablespoon olive oil and lemon juice sauce (or light vinaigrette of choice)
- 1 big egg

Preparation:

1. Cook bulgur wheat according to package directions.
2. While bulgur cooks, bring a pot of water to a simmer.
3. Crack the egg into a small bowl. Gently swirl the simmering water to form a vortex and carefully drop the egg into the center.
4. Poach the egg for 4-5 minutes, for a runny yolk, or longer for a firmer yolk.
5. In a bowl, mix cooked bulgur wheat, cucumber, tomato, and parsley.
6. Top with the cooked egg and drizzle with dressing.

7. Sprinkle with feta cheese (if using) before serving.

Nutritional Value(per serving):

- Calories: 350

- Protein: 18g

- Fat: 10g

- Carbohydrates: 40g

Cooking Time: 10 minutes

Serving: 1

Lamb Chop with Sweet Potato Mash & Vegetables

Ingredients:

Lamb Chop:

- 1 bone-in lamb chop (4-5 oz)

- 1/2 tablespoon olive oil

- Salt and pepper to taste

Sweet Potato Mash:

- 1 small sweet potato, peeled and diced

- 1 tablespoon milk (or water)

- Salt and pepper to taste

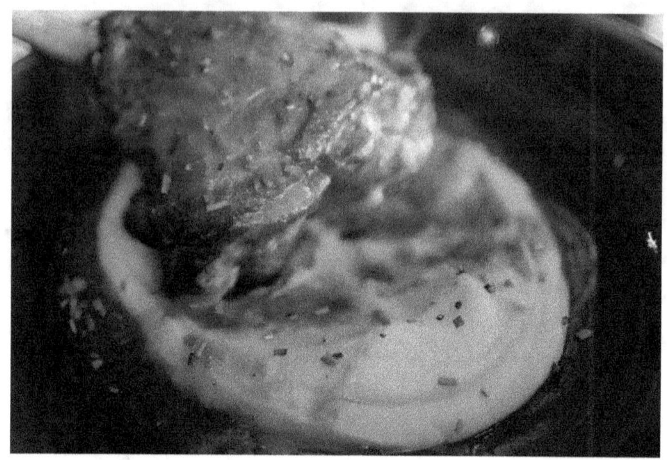

Vegetables:

- 1/2 cup steamed asparagus spears

- 1/4 cup cherry tomatoes, halved

Preparation:

1. Preheat your oven to 400°F (200°C).

2. Place diced sweet potato in a small pot, top with water, and bring to a boil. Then reduce heat and simmer for 10-15 minutes or until tender.

3. While sweet potato cooks, heat olive oil in a pan over medium heat. Apply salt and pepper to the lamb chop.

4. Sear lamb chop for 2-3 minutes per side.

5. Transfer lamb chop to a baking dish and place in the preheated oven for 10-12 minutes, or until cooked through (desired core temperature for lamb is 145°F (63°C) for medium-rare).

6. While the lamb cooks, steam the asparagus according to package directions.

7. Drain cooked sweet potato and mash with milk (or water) until smooth. Add salt and pepper to taste. Serve the lamb chop with mash potato and vegetable

Nutritional Value (per serving):

- Calories: 500

- Protein: 35g

- Fat: 25g

- Carbohydrates: 35g

Cooking Time: 45 minutes

Serving 1

Turkey Meatloaf with Mashed Cauliflower

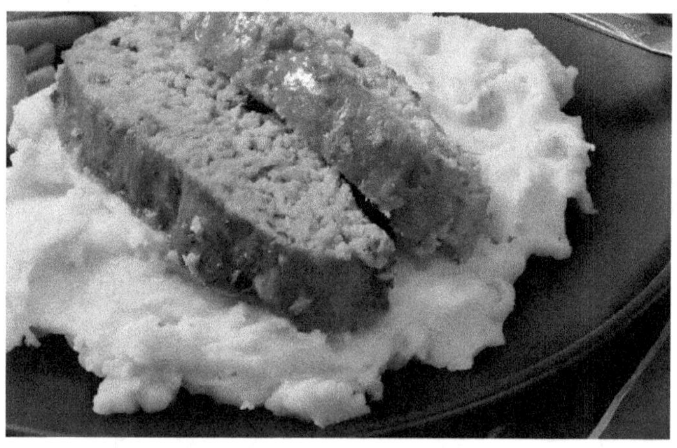

Ingredients:

Meatloaf:

- 1 pound ground turkey

- 1/2 cup chopped onion

- 1/4 cup chopped celery

- 1/4 cup panko breadcrumbs

- 1 egg, beaten

- 1 tablespoon ketchup

- 1 tablespoon Worcestershire sauce

- 1/2 teaspoon dried thyme

- Salt and pepper to taste

Mashed Cauliflower:

- 1 head cauliflower, chopped into florets

- 1/4 cup low-fat milk

- 1 tablespoon butter

- Salt and pepper to taste

Preparation:

1. Preheat your oven to 375°F (190°C). Lightly oil a baking dish.

2. In a large bowl, combine ground turkey, onion, celery, breadcrumbs, egg, ketchup, Worcestershire sauce, thyme, salt, and pepper. Mix well.

3. Form the mixture into a loaf form and set it in the prepared baking dish.

4. Bake for 30-35 minutes, or until cooked through (internal temperature should reach 165°F (74°C)).

5. While the meatloaf cooks, steam cauliflower florets until cooked, about 10-15 minutes.

6. Drain cauliflower and mash it with milk and butter until smooth. Season with salt and pepper. Serve your meatloaf with the mashed cauliflower.

Nutritional Value (per serving):

- Calories: 450
- Protein: 40g

- Fat: 15g
- Carbohydrates: 30g

Cooking Time: 45 minutes

Serving: 2

Chicken Stir-Fry with Brown Rice & Edamame

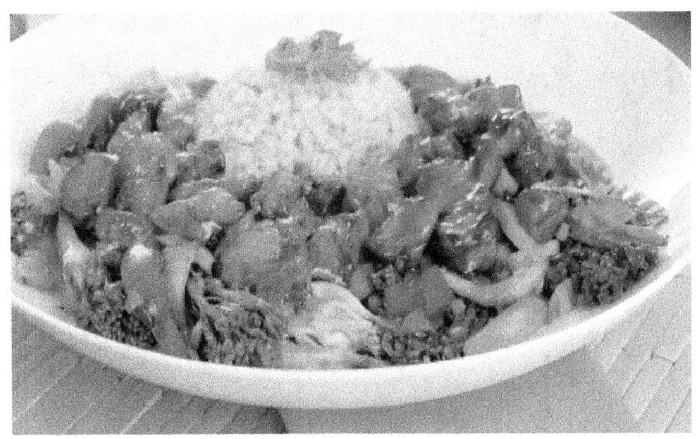

Ingredients:

Stir-Fry:

- 1 boneless, skinless chicken breast (4-5 oz), sliced
- 1/4 cup of olive oil

- 1/2 cup chopped broccoli florets

- 1/4 cup sliced red bell pepper

- 1/4 cup chopped snow peas

- 1 tablespoon soy sauce

- One tablespoon cornstarch mixed with two Tbsp water (cornstarch slurry)

- Salt and pepper to taste

Brown Rice: 1/2 cup cooked brown rice

Preparation:

1. Cook brown rice according to package guidelines while cooking.

2. Warm your olive oil in a large skillet or wok over medium-high heat.

3. Add chicken and sauté until browned and cooked through, about 5 minutes.

4. Add broccoli, red pepper, and snow peas, and simmer for 3-4 minutes, or until tender-crisp.

5. In a small bowl, stir together soy sauce and cornstarch slurry.

6. Add the sauce mixture into the skillet with the chicken and vegetables and allow to cook for 1 minute, or until the sauce thickens.

7. Add salt and pepper to taste.

Nutritional Value (per serving):

- Calories: 400
- Protein: 35g
- Fat: 10g
- Carbohydrates: 35g

Cooking Time: 30 minutes

Serving: 1

Lentil Shepherd's Pie with Creamy Mashed Potatoes

Ingredients:

Lentil Filling:

- 1 tablespoon olive oil

- 1 medium onion, chopped

- 2 cloves garlic, minced

- 1 carrot, diced

- 1 celery stalk, chopped

- 1 cup brown lentils, washed

- 4 cups low-sodium vegetable broth

- 1 can (14.5 oz) diced tomatoes, undrained

- 1/2 teaspoon dried thyme

- 1/4 teaspoon dried rosemary

- Salt and pepper to taste

Mashed Potatoes:

- 2 medium potatoes, peeled and diced

- 1/4 cup low-fat milk

- 1 tablespoon butter

- Salt and pepper to taste

Preparation:

1. Preheat your oven to 400°F (200°C).
   Lightly oil a baking dish.

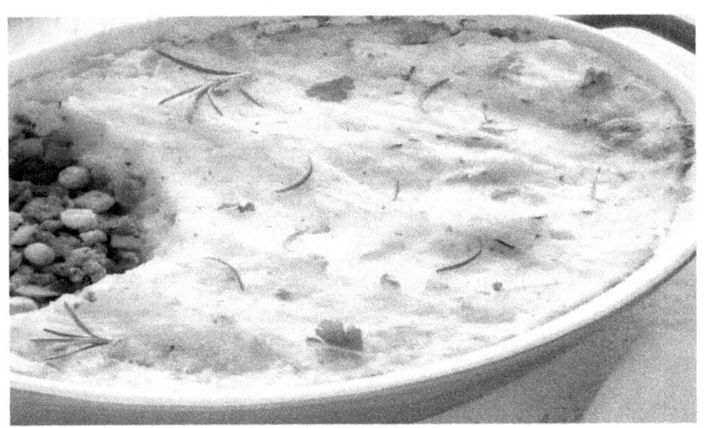

2. Heat your olive oil in a big pot over
   medium heat. Put onion, garlic, carrot,
   and celery, simmer until softened,
   about 5 minutes.
3. Add lentils, vegetable broth, diced
   tomatoes, thyme, and rosemary.
   Season with salt and pepper.
4. Bring to a boil, then decrease heat and
   simmer for 20-25 minutes, or until
   lentils are cooked.

5. While the lentil mixture simmers, cook potatoes in a pot of boiling water until cooked, about 15-20 minutes.

6. Drain potatoes and mash them with milk and butter until smooth. Season with salt and pepper.

7. Spoon the lentil mixture into the prepared baking dish. Top with mashed potatoes, spreading evenly.

8. Bake for 15-20 minutes until heated through and the top is softly golden brown.

Nutritional Value (per serving):
- Calories: 450
- Protein: 25g
- Fat: 12g
- Carbohydrates: 50g

Cooking Time: 45 minutes

Serving: 2

Chapter 4: Poultry and Seafoods

Lean Meat and Poultry Diets Recipes:

Grilled Chicken Caesar Salad with Whole Grain Croutons

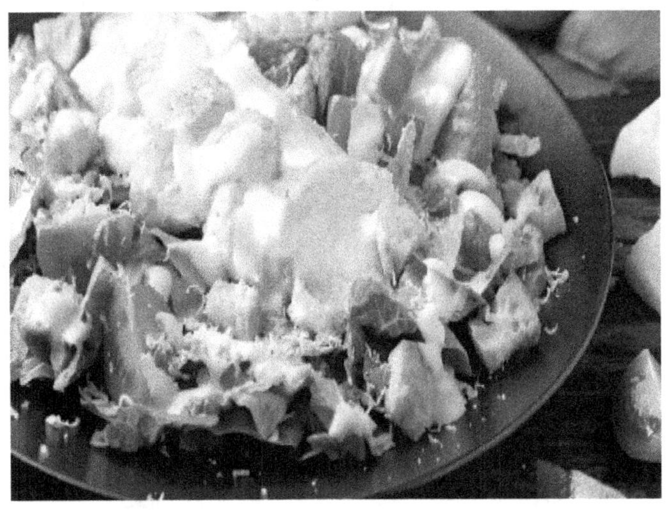

Ingredients:

- 6 oz grilled chicken breast, sliced
- 2 cups romaine lettuce, chopped
- 1/2 cup cherry tomatoes, split

- 1/4 cup whole grain croutons
- 2 tablespoons Caesar sauce (low-fat)
- 1 tablespoon grated Parmesan cheese

Preparation:

1. Firstly grill your chicken breast until fully cooked, then slice.
2. In a large bowl, toss together romaine salad, cherry tomatoes, and grilled chicken slices.
3. Add whole-grain croutons to the salad.
4. Drizzle Caesar dressing over the salad and toss to coat equally.
5. Sprinkle chopped Parmesan cheese on top before serving.

Nutritional Value (Approx.):

- Protein: 30g
- Fiber: 4g
- Calories: 350

Turkey and Vegetable Skewers with Quinoa

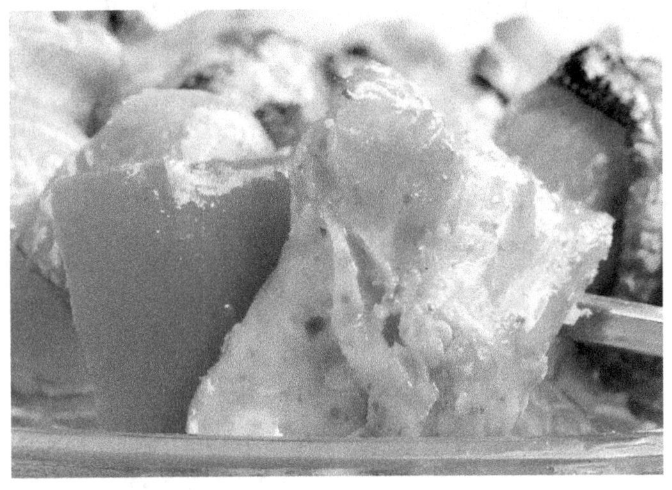

Ingredients:

- 8 oz lean ground turkey
- 1/2 cup bell peppers, diced
- 1/2 cup zucchini, sliced
- 1/2 cup red onion, cut into chunks
- 1 cup cooked quinoa

- 1 tablespoon olive oil

- 1 teaspoon smoked pepper

- Salt and pepper to taste

- Fresh parsley for garnish

Preparation:

1. Set your grill or oven to medium-high heat.

2. In a bowl, mix ground turkey with smoked paprika, salt, and pepper. Form the mixture into small meatballs.

3. Thread meatballs onto skewers alternate with diced bell peppers, zucchini, and red onion.

4. Grill or bake the skewers for about 12-15 minutes or until the turkey is fully cooked.

5. While the skewers are cooking, toss the cooked quinoa with olive oil.

6. Serve the turkey and veggie skewers over a bed of quinoa, garnished with fresh parsley.

Nutritional Value (Approx.):

- Protein: 28g
- Fiber: 6g
- Calories: 400

Cooking Time: 20 minutes
Serving Size: 1 serving

Spanish pork shoulder steaks with beans

Ingredients:

- Three garlic cloves crushed, 2 sliced
- 2 tbsp rapeseed oil
- 4 tsp smoked pepper
- 4 lean pork shoulder steaks (525g), shaved of any fat
- 2 large onions, split and sliced

- 6 carrots, diced

- 2 tbsp sherry vinegar

- 2 red peppers, deseeded and chopped

- 1 tbsp vegetable bouillon powder, made up to 500ml with hot water

- Three rosemary sprigs, leaves picked and finely chopped

- 200g cherry tomatoes

- 2 tbsp tomato purée

- 2 x 400g cans butter beans, drained

- ⅓ x 30g pack parsley, chopped

- squeeze of lemon (optional)

Preparation:

1. Mix the crushed garlic, 1 tbsp of the oil and 1 tsp smoked paprika together in a small dish and turn the pork steaks over in the mix to coat them on both sides.

2. Heat a big non-stick frying pan and fry the pork for about 4 mins on each side to part-cook and brown them, then remove them from the pan.

3. Add the rest of the oil to the pan and fry the onions, carrots, and sliced garlic, turning frequently for 10 mins until the veg starts to caramelize a little.

4. Pour in the sherry vinegar, letting it sizzle in the heat, then add the peppers, bouillon, rosemary, any juices left in the dish from the pork, the cherry tomatoes, tomato purée, remaining 3 tsp paprika, and beans.

5. Lay the pork steaks on top, then cover the pan and cook for 20 minutes until the pork and veggies are tender.

6. Remove the pork from the pan, stir in the parsley and a squeeze of lemon juice, if using. Enjoy

Nutritional value per serving:

- Calories:454
- Carbs: 35g
- Fiber: 17g
- Protein: 39g

Cooking Time: 40 min

serving: 4

Thai beef stir-fry

Ingredients:

- 2 tbsp vegetable oil
- 400g meat strips, or steak cut into thin strips
- 1 red chili, deseeded and finely chopped
- 2 tbsp oyster sauce

- handful basil leaves

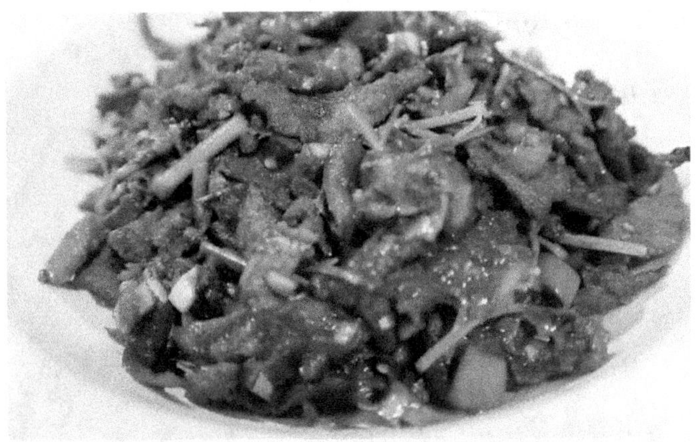

Preparation:

1. Heat your wok or big frying pan until smoking hot then pour in oil and swirl around the pan, tip in the beef strips and chili.

2. Cook and frequently stir until the meat is lightly browned, about 3 mins, then pour over the oyster sauce.

3. Allow to cook until cooked through and the sauce coats the meat. Then

stir in the basil leaves and serve with brown rice.

Nutritional value per serving:

- Calories:178
- Carbs:1g
- Fiber 0g
- Protein 22g

Cooking Time:5 min

Serving: 4

Beef bourguignon with celeriac mash

Ingredients:

- 1 tbsp goose fat
- 600g shin beef, cut into large chunks
- 100g smoked streaky bacon, sliced
- 350g shallot or pearl onions, chopped
- 250g chestnut mushrooms (about 20)

- 2 garlic cloves, sliced

- 1 bouquet garni

- 1 tbsp tomato purée

- 750ml bottle of red wine, Burgundy is good

For the celeriac mash:

- 600g (about 1) celeriac

- 2 tbsp olive oil, plus a glug

- 1 or 2 rosemary and thyme leaves

- 2 bay leaves

- 4 cardamom pods

Preparation:

1. Warm your big casserole pan and add 1 tbsp goose fat.

2. After Seasoning your shin, fry until golden brown, about 3-5 mins, then turn over and fry the other side until the meat is cooked all over, adding more fat if necessary. repeat in 2-3

steps, transferring the meat to a colander set over a bowl when browned.

3. In the same pan, fry streaky bacon, peeled shallots or pearl onions, chestnut mushrooms, 2 sliced garlic cloves, and 1 bouquet garni until lightly browned.

4. Mix in 1 tbsp tomato purée and cook for a few minutes, turning the mixture. This improves the bourguignon and makes a great base for the stew. Then take back the beef and any drained juices to the pan and stir through.

5. Pour over a red wine and about 100ml water so the meat bobs up from the liquid, but isn't completely covered.

6. Carry to a boil and use a spoon to scrape the caramelized cooking juices from the bottom of the pan – this will give the stew more taste.

7. Heat oven to 150 F/ 130C

8. *Make a cartouche:* tear off a square of foil slightly larger than the casserole, arrange it in the pan so it covers the top of the stew, and trim away any extra foil. Cook for 3 hrs.

9. If the sauce looks watery, remove the meat and veggies with a slotted spoon, and set aside. Cook the sauce over high heat for a few minutes until the sauce has thickened a little, then take back the beef and veggies to the pan.

10. *To make the celeriac mash:* peel 600g of celeriac and cut into cubes.

Heat 2 tbsp olive oil in a big frying pan. Pour in the celeriac and fry for 5 mins until it turns golden. Season well with salt and pepper.

11. Stir in your sprigs of rosemary and thyme, bay leaves, and cardamom pods, then pour over 200 ml water, enough to nearly cover the celeriac. Turn the heat to low, slightly cover the pan, and leave to simmer for 25-30 mins.

12. After 25-30 mins, the celeriac should be soft and most of the water will have drained. Drain away any leftover water, then remove the herb sprigs, bay, and cardamom pods.

13. Lightly crush with a potato masher, then finish with a glug of olive oil and season to taste.

14. Spoon the beef bourguignon into serving bowls and put a large spoonful of the celeriac mash on top.

15. Decorate with one of the bay leaves, if you like and enjoy.

Nutritional value per serving:

- Calories: 571
- Carbs: 16g, fiber: 8g
- Protein: 42g

Cook: 3 hr 15 minutes

Serve: 4

Creamy spinach chicken

One-Pan Creamy Chicken and Spinach (Quick and Easy)

Ingredients:

- 2 tablespoons olive oil

- 1.5 pounds boneless, skinless chicken breasts or chicken tenderloins (cut into bite-sized pieces)
- 2 tablespoons butter
- 1/3 cup finely diced onion
- 3 cloves garlic, minced
- 1/2 teaspoon crushed red pepper flakes (optional)
- 1 cup heavy cream
- 1 cup chicken broth
- 2 tablespoons chopped sun-dried tomatoes (optional)
- 2 ounces cream cheese, softened
- 1/2 cup grated Parmesan cheese
- 3 cups fresh spinach leaves, chopped (or 5 oz frozen spinach, thawed and squeezed dry)
- Salt and freshly ground black pepper to taste

- Chopped fresh basil (optional, for garnish)

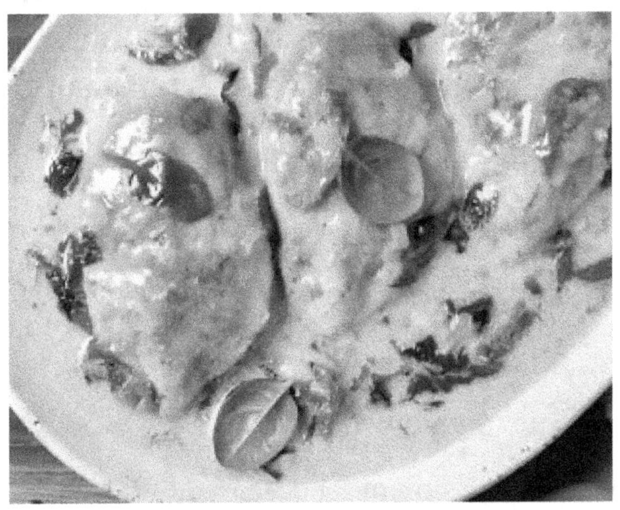

Preparation:

1. Warm your olive oil in a big skillet over medium heat. Apply salt and pepper to the chicken. Put the chicken in the pan and cook for 5-7 minutes or until golden brown and cooked through. Take away the chicken from the pan and set aside.

2. Dissolve the butter in the same pan over medium heat. Put onion and garlic and cook until softened, about 5 minutes. Mix in crushed red pepper flakes (if using).

3. Pour in heavy cream and chicken stock. Carry to a boil and cook for 2-3 minutes, or until slightly thickened.

4. Stir in chopped sun-dried tomatoes (if using), cream cheese, and Parmesan cheese. Allow to cook until the cheese is melted and the sauce is smooth.

5. Put the cooked chicken back into the pan and stir to coat in the sauce.

6. Finally, stir in the spinach and cook until wilted, about 1-2 minutes (or until heated through for frozen spinach).

7. Season with extra salt and pepper to taste. Garnish with chopped fresh basil (optional) before serving.

Nutritional value per serving:

- Calories: 500-550

- Protein: 30-35g

- Fat: 25-30g

- Carbs: 20-25g

Cooking Time: 30-minute

Serves: 4

Creamy Spinach Chicken with Lemon and Capers (Light and Zesty)

Ingredients:

- 2 tablespoons olive oil

- One pound boneless, skinless chicken breasts (thinly sliced or pounded thin)

- 1/2 teaspoon salt

- 1/4 teaspoon black pepper

- 1 tablespoon all-purpose flour

- 2 tablespoons butter

- 1 onion, chopped

- 2 cloves garlic, minced

- 1/2 cup dry white wine

- 1 cup chicken broth

- 1/2 cup heavy cream

- 2 tablespoons lemon juice

- 2 tablespoons capers, drained

- 4 cups fresh spinach leaves, chopped (or 6 oz frozen spinach, thawed and squeezed dry)

- 1/4 cup grated Parmesan cheese

- Chopped fresh parsley (optional, for garnish)

Preparation:

1. Season chicken breasts with salt and pepper. Dredge in flour to coat lightly.

2. Heat olive oil in a big skillet over medium heat. Add chicken and cook for 3-4 minutes per side or until golden brown and cooked through. Take away the chicken from the pan and set aside.

3. Dissolve the butter in the same pan over medium heat. Put onion and garlic and cook until softened, about 5 minutes.

4. Put white wine and pick up any browned bits from the bottom of the pan. Let the wine boil for a minute or two to reduce slightly.

5. Put in the chicken broth and bring to a simmer. Allow to cook for 5 minutes, or until the liquid drops slightly.

6. Stir in heavy cream, lemon juice, and capers. Leave the sauce to cook for a minute or two.

7. Put the cooked chicken back into the pan and stir to coat in the sauce.

8. Finally, stir in the spinach and cook until wilted, about 1-2 minutes (or until heated through for frozen spinach).

9. Stir in grated Parmesan cheese and season with extra salt and pepper to taste.

10. Garnish with chopped fresh parsley (optional) before serving.

Nutritional value per serving:

- Calories: 450-500
- Protein: 30-35g
- Fat: 20-25g
- Carbs: 30-35g

Cooking Time: 40 minutes

Serving: 4

Creamy Dijon Chicken with Spinach and Mushrooms (Rich and Flavorful)

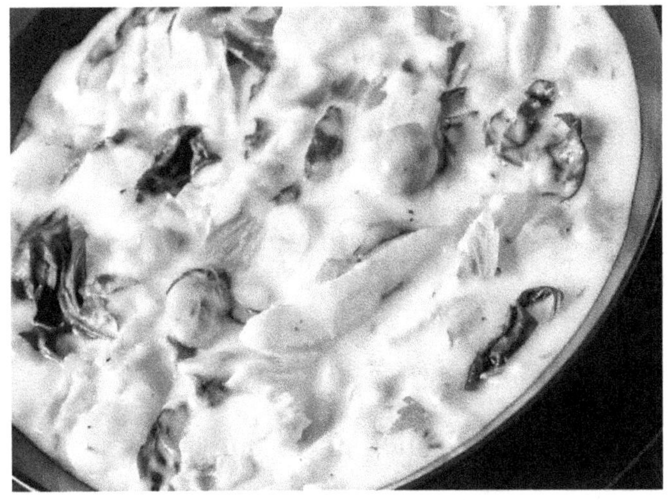

Ingredients:

- 2 tablespoons olive oil
- 1 pound boneless, skinless chicken breasts (cut into bite-sized pieces)
- 1/2 teaspoon salt

- 1/4 teaspoon of black pepper
- 1/2 teaspoon paprika
- 1 tablespoon Dijon mustard
- 2 tablespoons butter
- 1 onion, chopped
- 8 ounces mushrooms, sliced
- 2 cloves garlic, minced
- 1/2 cup dry white wine (optional)
- 1 cup chicken broth
- 1 cup thick cream
- 3 cups fresh spinach leaves, chopped (or 5 oz frozen spinach, thawed and squeezed dry)
- 1/4 cup grated Parmesan cheese
- Chopped fresh onions (optional, for garnish)

Preparation:

1. Season chicken bits with salt, pepper, and paprika. In a bowl, toss chicken with Dijon mustard to coat evenly.

2. Heat olive oil in a big skillet over medium heat. Add chicken and cook for 5-7 minutes or until golden brown and cooked through. Take away the chicken from the pan and set aside.

3. Dissolve the butter in the same pan over medium heat. Put onion and mushrooms and cook until softened, about 5 minutes. Mix in garlic and cook for another minute. Then pour in white wine (if using) and scrape up any burnt bits from the bottom of the pan. Leave the wine to boil for a minute or two to reduce slightly.

4. Put the chicken broth and bring to a simmer. Allow to cook for 5 minutes, or until the liquid drops slightly.

5. Mix in heavy cream. Leave the sauce to cook for a minute or two.

6. Put the cooked chicken back into the pan and stir to coat in the sauce.

7. Finally, stir in the spinach and cook until wilted, about 1-2 minutes (or until heated through for frozen spinach).

8. Mix in the grated Parmesan cheese and season with extra salt and pepper to taste.

9. Garnish with chopped fresh chives (optional) and serve quickly.

Nutritional Value Serve:

- Calories: 500-550
- Protein: 35-40g

- Fat: 30-35g
- Carbs: 25-30g

Cooking Time: 45 minutes

Serving: 4

Chicken jalfrezi

Ingredients:

For the sauce:

- ½ large onion, roughly chopped
- 2 garlic cloves, chopped
- 1 green chili, finely chopped
- vegetable oil, for frying
- 400g can plum tomatoes
- 1 tbsp ground coriander
- 1 tbsp ground cumin
- 1 tsp turmeric

For the meat & veg:

- 2-3 chicken breasts, diced
- 1 tsp ground cumin

- 1 tsp ground coriander
- 1 tsp turmeric
- ½ large onion, sliced
- 1 red pepper, chopped
- 2 red chilies, finely chopped (optional)
- 2 tsp garam masala
- handful of fresh, chopped coriander leaves
- cooked basmati rice or naan bread to serve

Preparation:

1. Coat the chicken breasts with 1 tsp cumin, 1 tsp coriander, and 1 tsp turmeric then leave it to marinate in the fridge while you make the sauce.

2. ***To make the sauce:*** fry your onion, garlic cloves, and green chili in a

large pan with a little vegetable oil, for around 5 mins, until browned.

3. Put 300ml water in the onion mixture and simmer for around 20 minutes.

4. Then put plum tomatoes in a food processor and give them a good whizz (aim for a smooth consistency).

5. Warm another large pan and gently fry 1 tbsp coriander, 1 tbsp cumin, and 1 tsp turmeric in a splash of oil for about a minute. Put the tomatoes in this pan and simmer for around 10 minutes. Then whizz your onion mixture in the food processor and add it to the spiced tomato sauce. add a little salt and pepper and stir, then simmer for 20 minutes. You can make large batches of this sauce and freeze it for later use if desired.

6. Then fry the marinated chicken in vegetable oil and stir continuously. After a few minutes, turn down the heat and put the remaining ½ sliced onion, 1 chopped red pepper, and 2 finely chopped red chilies and stir until the onions and pepper soften.

7. Pour your sauce onto the cooked chicken and simmer for around 10-20 minutes, adding a splash of water if it gets too thick.

8. Before dishing out, stir in 2 tsp garam masala and a handful of chopped coriander leaves. Enjoy with basmati rice or naan bread.

Nutritional value per serving:

- calories: 252, carbs: 11g
- fiber: 5g
- Protein: 30g

Cook:1hr

Serving: 4

Fish and Seafoods:

Lobster with Thermidor Butter

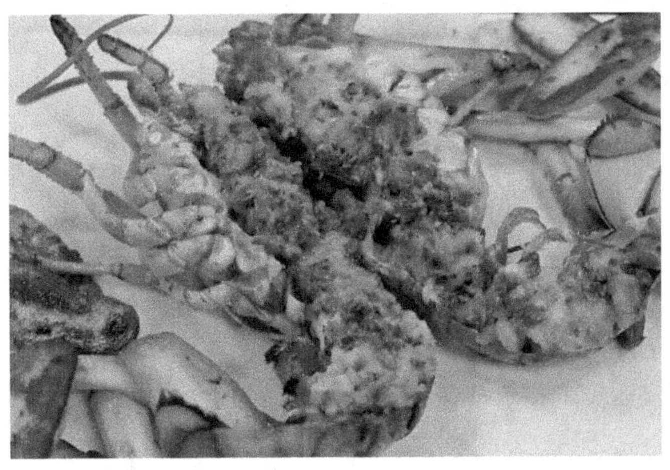

Ingredients:

Lobster:

- 1 (1-1/2 pound) cooked lobster, halved and cleaned

Thermidor Butter:

- 2 tablespoons butter, softened

- 1 shallot, finely chopped

- 1 tablespoon Cognac (optional)

- 1/4 cup dry white wine

- 1/4 cup heavy cream

- 1 tablespoon Dijon mustard

- 1/4 cup grated Parmesan cheese

- 1 egg yolk

- Pinch of cayenne pepper

- Salt and pepper to taste

- ***Garnish: Fresh chopped parsley (optional)***

Preparation:

1. ***Make the Thermidor Butter:*** In a small bowl, cream together the softened butter and Dijon mustard. Stir in the shallot and cayenne pepper.

2. In a small saucepan, heat the Cognac (if using) over medium heat until

almost simmering. Carefully ignite the Cognac with a match (with appropriate ventilation) and let the flame burn out.

3. Put the white wine in the pan and simmer until reduced by half.

4. Stir in the heavy cream and heat for 1 minute. Remove from heat and mix in the egg yolk and Parmesan cheese. Put a little salt and pepper to taste.

5. ***Prepare the Lobster:*** Preheat the broiler to high. Arrange the lobster halves on a baking sheet, cut side up. Spoon the Thermidor butter evenly over the lobster flesh.

6. Broil for 3-4 minutes, or until the topping is bubbling and golden brown.

7. *Serve:* Garnish with fresh parsley (optional) and enjoy immediately.

Nutritional Information (per serving):

- Calories: 650
- Protein: 50g
- Fat: 45g
- Carbohydrates: 10g

Cooking Time:30 minutes

Serves 1

Clams with Sherry & Serrano Ham

Ingredients:

Clams:

- 1 pound fresh clams, washed and debearded
- 1/2 cup dry white wine
- 1/4 cup water

Sauté:

- 2 tablespoons olive oil

- 1 shallot, finely chopped
- 2 minced garlic cloves
- 1/4 cup chopped Serrano ham
- 1/4 cup dry sherry
- 1/4 cup chopped fresh parsley
- Salt and pepper to taste

Preparation:

1. Combine the white wine, water, and clams in a large pot. Cover and carry to a boil over high heat. Allow to cook for 5-7 minutes, or until the clams open. Discard any unopened clams.

2. While the clams simmer, heat olive oil in a large skillet over medium heat. Add shallot and garlic, and sauté until softened, about 2 minutes.

3. Stir in the chopped Serrano ham and heat for a further minute.

4. Pour in the sherry and simmer for another minute, scraping up any browned bits from the bottom of the pan.

5. Add the cooked clams and their broth to the skillet and simmer for 2-3 minutes, or until heated through.

6. Season with salt and pepper to taste.

7. *Serve:* Sprinkle with fresh parsley and serve with crusty bread for dipping in the delightful broth.

Nutritional Information (per serving):

- Calories: 350
- Protein: 30g
- Fat: 15g
- Carbohydrates: 15g

Cooking Time: 20 minutes

Serving: 2

Stir-fry Prawns with Peppers & Spinach

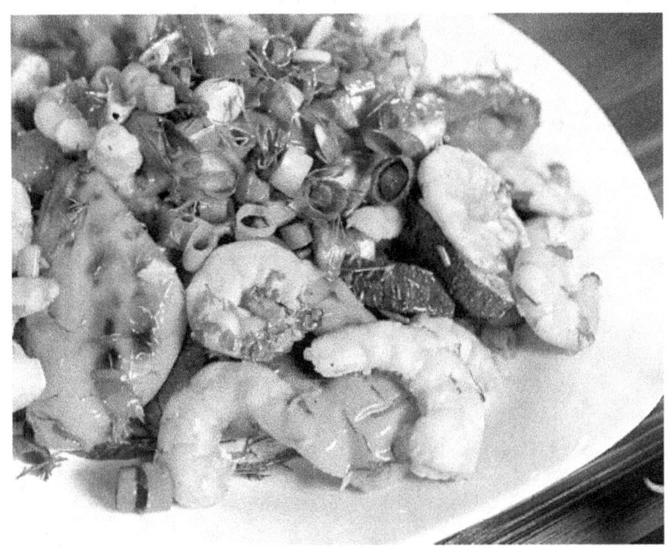

Ingredients:

Stir-fry:

- 1/2 pound shelled and deveined prawns
- 1/4 cup of olive oil
- 1/2 red bell pepper, sliced
- 1/2 yellow bell pepper, sliced
- 1/4 cup chopped onion

- 1 cup fresh spinach

Stir-fry:

- 1 tablespoon soy sauce

- One tablespoon cornstarch mixed with

- Two tablespoons water (cornstarch slurry)

- Salt and pepper to taste

- ***Garnish:*** Chopped scallions (optional)

Preparation:

1. In a small bowl, whisk together the soy sauce and cornstarch slurry.

2. Warm your olive oil in a large skillet or wok over medium-high heat. Put prawns and cook for 2-3 minutes per side or until pink and opaque. Take them out from the pan and set aside.

3. Add the bell peppers and onion to the pan, and simmer for 3-4 minutes, or until softened.

4. Stir in the spinach and simmer for another minute, or until wilted.

5. Pour the soy sauce mixture into the pan and bring to a simmer. Allow to cook for 1 more minute, or until the sauce thickens.

6. Return the cooked prawns to the pan and toss to coat with the sauce.

7. Season with salt and pepper to taste.

8. *Serve:* Serve immediately over rice or noodles, topped with sliced scallions (optional).

Nutritional Value (per serving):

- Calories: 400
- Protein: 35g
- Fat: 15g

- Carbohydrates: 20g

Cooking Time: 15 minutes

Serving: 1

<u>Sweet Hot Prawn & Pineapple Curry</u>

Ingredients:

- 1 tablespoon vegetable oil
- 1 onion, chopped
- Two cloves garlic, minced
- 1 tablespoon grated ginger
- 1 red chili pepper, deseeded and finely chopped (modify according to spice preference)
- 1 tablespoon curry powder
- 1/2 teaspoon turmeric powder
- Canned diced tomatoes, 1 (15 ounces) can (undrained)

- 1 (13.5 oz) can light coconut milk

- 1/2 cup chopped fresh pineapple

- 1 pound shelled and deveined prawns

- 1 tablespoon fish sauce (optional)

- 1 tablespoon lime juice

- Freshly ground black pepper to taste and a little salt

- *Garnish:* Chopped fresh cilantro (optional)

- Cooked rice or noodles (for serving)

Preparation:

1. Warm your vegetable oil in a big pot or Dutch oven over medium heat. Put onion and simmer until softened for about 5 minutes.

2. Stir in garlic, ginger, and chili pepper, and simmer for an additional minute, until fragrant.

3. Add curry powder and turmeric powder, and simmer for another minute, stirring regularly to unleash the flavors.

4. Put your diced tomatoes and coconut milk. Then carry to a simmer and cook for 5 minutes.

5. Stir in the chopped pineapple and simmer for another 5 minutes, or until the pineapple softens slightly.

6. Add the prawns and boil for 3-4 minutes or until pink and opaque.

7. (Optional) Stir in fish sauce and lime juice. Put freshly ground black pepper to taste and a little salt.

8. Serve: Garnish with chopped fresh cilantro (optional) and serve hot cooked rice or noodles.

Nutritional Value (per serving):

- Calories: 450
- Protein: 40g
- Fat: 20g
- Carbohydrates: 30g

Cooking Time: 30 minutes

Serving: 2

Curry Coconut Fish Parcels

Ingredients:

Fish Parcel:

- 4 oz white fish filet (such as cod, tilapia, or halibut)
- 1/4 cup chopped red bell pepper
- 1/4 cup chopped green beans
- 1 tablespoon chopped fresh parsley
- Salt and pepper to taste

Curry Sauce:

- 1/2 tbsp vegetable oil

- 1/2 shallot, finely chopped

- 1 clove garlic, minced

- 1/2 teaspoon curry powder

- 1/4 cup light coconut milk

- 1 tablespoon fish sauce (optional)

- 1 tablespoon lime juice

- Salt and pepper to taste

- *Garnish*: Chopped fresh cilantro (optional)

- Cooked rice or noodles (for serving)

Preparation:

1. Preheat your oven to 400°F (200°C). Then line a baking sheet with parchment paper.

2. ***Prepare the Fish Parcel:*** Place the fish filet in the center of a large piece of parchment paper. Season with salt and pepper.

3. Top the fish with chopped red bell pepper, green beans, and fresh parsley.

4. Fold the parchment paper over the fish and vegetables, making a sealed parcel.

5. ***Make the Curry Sauce:*** In a small saucepan, heat oil over medium heat. Add shallot and garlic, and sauté until softened, about 1 minute.

6. Stir in curry powder, and simmer for an additional minute, until aromatic.

7. Pour in the coconut milk, fish sauce (optional), and lime juice. carry to a simmer and cook for 2 minutes.

8. Carefully transfer the fish bundle to the prepared baking sheet. Pour a few teaspoons of the curry sauce around the bottom of the packet.

9. Bake for 12-15 minutes, or until the fish is cooked through and flakes readily with a fork.

10. ***Serve:*** Carefully open the parchment paper packet and spread the remaining curry sauce over the fish and vegetables. Garnish with chopped fresh cilantro (optional) and serve hot cooked rice or noodles.

Nutritional Value (per serving):

- Calories: 400
- Protein: 35g
- Fat: 15g
- Carbohydrates: 30g

Cooking Time: 25 minutes

Serving: 1

Creamy Crab Curry

Ingredients:

Curry:

- 1 tablespoon vegetable oil
- 1 onion, chopped
- 2 minced garlic cloves
- 1 tablespoon grated ginger
- 1 tablespoon curry powder
- 1/2 teaspoon turmeric powder
- Canned diced tomatoes, 1 (15 ounces) can (undrained)
- 1 (13.5 oz) can light coconut milk
- 1 cup low-sodium chicken broth
- 1/2 cup sliced fresh green beans
- 8 oz cooked crabmeat (lump or shredded)
- 1 tablespoon fish sauce (optional)
- 1 tablespoon lime juice
- Freshly ground black pepper to taste and a little salt

Garnish:

- Chopped fresh cilantro (optional)
- Cooked rice or noodles (for serving)

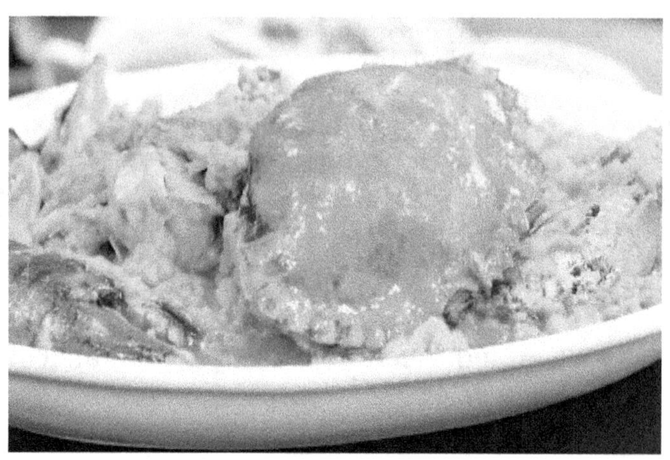

Preparation:

1. Heat vegetable oil in a big pot or Dutch oven over medium heat. Add onion and simmer until softened, about 5 minutes.

2. Stir in garlic and ginger, and simmer for an additional minute, until fragrant.

3. Add curry powder and turmeric powder, and simmer for another

minute, stirring regularly to unleash the flavors.

4. Pour in your coconut milk, diced tomatoes, and chicken broth. Carry to a simmer and cook for 10 minutes.

5. Add the chopped green beans and cook for another 5 minutes, or until tender-crisp.

6. Gently whisk in the cooked crabmeat.

7. (Optional) Stir in fish sauce and lime juice. Season with freshly ground black pepper to taste and a little salt.

8. *Serve:* Garnish with chopped fresh cilantro (optional) and serve hot cooked rice or noodles.

Nutritional Value (per serving):

- Calories: 500
- Protein: 45g
- Fat: 25g

- Carbohydrates: 35g

Cooking Time: 40 minutes

Serving: 2

Curried Cod with Roasted Vegetables

Ingredients:

fish:

- 1 fish filet (4-5 oz)
- 1/4 cup of olive oil
- 1/2 teaspoon curry powder
- Salt and pepper to taste

Roasted Vegetables:

- 1/2 cup chopped broccoli florets
- 1/4 cup cherry tomatoes, halved
- 1/4 cup of olive oil
- Salt and pepper to taste

Curry Sauce:

- 1/2 cup low-sodium vegetable broth

- 1 tablespoon chopped onion

- 1 clove garlic, minced

- 1/2 teaspoon curry powder

- 1/4 cup light coconut milk

- One tablespoon cornstarch mixed with two tablespoons water (cornstarch slurry)

- Salt and pepper to taste

Preparation:

1. Preheat your oven to 400°F (200°C). Then line a baking sheet with parchment paper.

2. ***To Roast Vegetable:*** Toss broccoli florets and cherry tomatoes with olive oil, salt, and pepper and stretch them on the prepared baking sheet.

3. Roast the vegetables for 15-20 minutes, or until tender-crisp.

4. While the vegetables roast, pat the cod filet dry and season with curry powder, salt, and pepper.

5. Heat the remaining tablespoon of olive oil in a large skillet over medium heat. Add the fish filet and heat for 5-7 minutes per side, or until cooked through and flakes easily with a fork.

6. ***Make the Curry Sauce:*** In a small saucepan, heat vegetable broth over medium heat. Put onion and garlic, and sauté until softened, about 2 minutes.

7. Stir in the remaining 1/2 teaspoon curry powder and simmer for an additional minute.

8. Put your coconut milk and bring to a simmer.

9. Whisk in the cornstarch slurry and heat for 1 minute, or until the sauce thickens. Add salt and pepper to taste.

10. *Serve:* Plate the roasted veggies, top with the cooked cod filet, then ladle the curry sauce over the top.

Nutritional Value (per serving):

- Calories: 400
- Protein: 35g
- Fat: 15g
- Carbohydrates: 30g

Cooking Time: 45 minutes

Serving: 1

Harissa Fish with Bulgur Salad

Ingredients:

Fish:

- 1 boneless, skinless white fish filet (4-5 oz)

- 1/4 cup of olive oil

- 1/2 teaspoon harissa paste

- Salt and pepper to taste

Bulgur Salad:

- 1/4 cup bulgur wheat

- 1/2 cucumber, deseeded and finely chopped

- 1/4 cup cherry tomatoes, quartered

- 2 tablespoons crumbled feta cheese (optional)

- 1 tablespoon chopped fresh parsley

- 1/4 cup of olive oil

- 1 tablespoon lemon juice

- Salt and pepper to taste

Preparation:

1. Preheat your oven to 400°F (200°C).

2. **Cook Bulgur:** In a small saucepan, combine bulgur wheat with 1/2 cup water. Carry to a boil, reduce heat,

cover, and simmer for 15 minutes, or until the bulgur is soft and fluffy. Fluff with a fork and leave aside to cool slightly.

3. While the bulgur cooks, pat the fish filet dry and season with salt and pepper.

4. In a small dish, combine the olive oil with the harissa paste. Brush the harissa mixture over the fish filet.

5. Put the fish on a baking sheet lined with parchment paper.

6. Bake for 15-20 minutes, or until cooked through and flakes readily with a fork.

7. ***Prepare the Bulgur Salad:*** In a bowl, combine chopped cucumber, cooked bulgur wheat, cherry tomatoes,

crumbled feta cheese (if using), and chopped parsley.

8. Drizzle with olive oil and lemon juice. Add salt and pepper to taste.

9. *Serve:* Plate the bulgur salad, top with the cooked harissa fish, and enjoy!

Nutritional Value (per serving):

- Calories: 400

- Protein: 30g

- Fat: 18g

- Carbohydrates: 30g

Cooking Time: 45 minutes

Serving: 1

Mediterranean Shrimp Scampi with Whole Wheat Pasta

Ingredients:

Shrimp Scampi:

- 1/2 pound shelled and deveined shrimp
- 1/4 cup of olive oil
- 2 minced garlic cloves
- 1/4 cup dry white wine (or chicken broth)
- 1/4 cup cherry tomatoes, halved
- 1 tablespoon chopped fresh parsley
- 1/4 teaspoon dried oregano
- Pinch of red pepper flakes (optional)
- Salt and pepper to taste
- *Pasta:* 1/2 cup cooked whole-wheat pasta
- *Garnish:* Chopped fresh basil (optional)

Preparation:

1. Cook whole-wheat pasta according to package directions while cooking, heat your olive oil in a large skillet

over medium heat. Put garlic and heat for 30 seconds, until fragrant.

2. Add shrimp and cook for 2-3 minutes per side or until pink and opaque.

3. Pour in white wine (or chicken broth), cherry tomatoes, parsley, oregano, and red pepper flakes (if using). Carry to a simmer and cook for 1 minute.

4. Season with salt and pepper to taste.

5. *Serve:* Drain the cooked pasta and add it to the skillet with the shrimp scampi sauce. Toss to blend.

6. Plate the spaghetti with shrimp and top with chopped fresh basil (optional).

Nutritional Value (per serving):

- Calories: 400
- Protein: 30g
- Fat: 15g

- Carbohydrates: 35g

Cooking Time: 20 minutes

Serving: 1

Shellfish, Orzo & Saffron Stew

Ingredients:

- 1/4 cup of olive oil

- 1 shallot, finely chopped

- 2 minced garlic cloves

- 1/2 teaspoon dried thyme

- 1/4 teaspoon ground fennel seed (optional)

- 1 cup chopped tomatoes (fresh or canned)

- 1 cup low-sodium chicken broth

- 1/4 cup dry white wine

- Pinch of saffron threads

- 1/2 cup orzo pasta

- 1/2 pound mussels, debearded and washed
- 1/4 pound shrimp, shelled and deveined (optional)
- 4-6 calamari rings, cleaned and sliced (optional)
- 1/4 cup chopped fresh parsley
- Salt and pepper to taste

Preparation:

1. Heat olive oil in a big pot or Dutch oven over medium heat. Add shallot and garlic, and sauté for 2 minutes, until softened.

2. Stir in thyme and fennel seed (if using), and simmer for a further minute, until aromatic.

3. Add diced tomatoes, chicken broth, white wine, and saffron threads. Carry to a simmer and cook for 10 minutes.

4. Add the orzo pasta and simmer for 5 minutes, or according to package recommendations for al dente.

5. Stir in mussels, shrimp (if used), and calamari (if used). Simmer for an additional 5-7 minutes, or until the mussels open and the shrimp and calamari are cooked through.

6. Discard any unopened mussels.

7. Stir in chopped parsley and season with salt and pepper to taste.

8. *Serve:* Enjoy the stew hot with fresh bread for dipping.

Nutritional Value (per serving):
- Calories: 450
- Protein: 40g
- Fat: 20g
- Carbohydrates: 35g

Cooking Time: 40 minutes

Serving: 2

Salmon & Prawns with Dill & Lime Aïoli

Ingredients:

Salmon & Prawns:

- 4 ounce salmon filet
- 1/2 tbsp olive oil
- Salt and pepper to taste
- 4-5 prawns, shelled and deveined (optional)

Dill & Lime Aïoli:

- 2 tablespoons mayonnaise (use good grade for maximum flavor)
- 1 tablespoon chopped fresh dill
- 1/2 teaspoon lime juice
- Pinch of garlic powder
- Salt and pepper to taste
- ***Garnish:*** Fresh dill sprig (optional)

Preparation:

1. Preheat your oven to 400°F (200°C).

2. Apply pepper and salt to the salmon filet and place it on a baking sheet lined with parchment paper.

3. (Optional) If using prawns, mix them with 1/2 tablespoon olive oil and season with salt and pepper. Arrange them on the baking sheet close to the salmon.

4. Allow to bake for 12-15 minutes, or until the salmon is cooked through and flakes easily with a fork, and the prawns are pink and opaque.

5. While the salmon and prawns cook, create the aïoli: In a small bowl, add mayonnaise, chopped dill, lime juice, garlic powder, salt, and pepper. Stir until well blended.

6. ***Serve:*** Plate the cooked salmon and prawns (if using). Dollop the dill & lime aïoli on the side and garnish with a fresh dill sprig (optional).

Nutritional Value (per serving):

- Calories: 450

- Protein: 40g

- Fat: 25g

- Carbohydrates: 5g

Cooking Time: 25 minutes

Serving: 1

Moroccan Seafood Tagine

Ingredients:

Tagine:

- 1/4 cup of olive oil

- 1 onion, chopped

- 2 minced garlic cloves

- 1 teaspoon ground ginger

- 1/2 teaspoon turmeric

- 1/2 teaspoon cinnamon

- 1/4 teaspoon cayenne pepper (modify according to spice preference)

- Canned diced tomatoes, 1 (15 ounces) can (undrained)

- 1 cup low-sodium chicken broth

- 1/2 cup chopped fresh cilantro

- 1/4 cup chopped fresh parsley

- Drain and rinse one 15-ounce can of chickpeas.

- 1 pound miscellaneous seafood (such as mussels, shrimp, scallops, or a combo)

- 1/2 cup green olives, pitted and halved (optional)

- Freshly ground black pepper to taste and a little salt

- ***Garnish:*** Chopped fresh parsley (optional)
- Crusty bread for serving

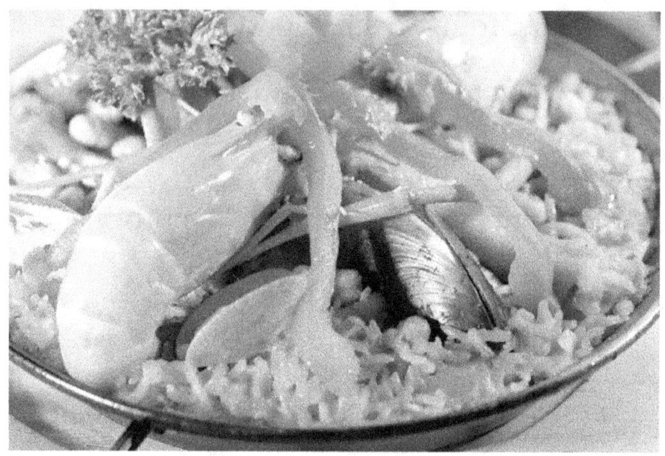

Preparation:

1. Heat olive oil in a large tagine or Dutch oven over medium heat. Add onion and simmer until softened, about 5 minutes.

2. Stir in garlic, ginger, turmeric, cinnamon, and cayenne pepper. Allow to cook for an additional minute, until fragrant.

3. Pour in the diced tomatoes, chicken broth, chopped cilantro, and parsley. Carry to a simmer and cook for 10 minutes.

4. (Optional) Stir in the drained and rinsed chickpeas.

5. Add the mixed seafood and simmer for a further 10-15 minutes, or until the mussels open and the shellfish is cooked thoroughly. Discard any unopened mussels.

6. Gently toss in the green olives (if using). Put freshly ground black pepper to taste and a little salt.

7. *Serve:* Serve the hot tagine with fresh bread for dipping. decorate with more chopped fresh parsley (optional).

Nutritional Value (per serving):

- Calories: 450

- Protein: 40g
- Fat: 20g
- Carbohydrates: 35g

Cooking Time: 1 hour 15 minutes

Serving: 4

Chapter 5: Plant-Based Protein Source

Lentil Shepherd's Pie with Creamy Cashew Mash

Ingredients:

Lentil Filling:

- 1 tablespoon olive oil
- 1 onion, chopped
- Two cloves garlic, minced
- 1 carrot, diced
- 1 celery stalk, diced
- 1 cup brown lentils, cleaned
- Undrained 1 (14.5 oz) can of diced tomatoes
- 1 cup low-sodium veggie broth
- 1/2 teaspoon dried thyme
- 1/4 teaspoon dried rosemary
- Salt and pepper to taste

Creamy Cashew Mash:

- 1 cup raw cashews, soaked for at least 2 hours or overnight
- 1/2 cup plain plant-based milk (such as almond or soy milk)
- 1 tablespoon healthy yeast (optional)
- Salt and pepper to taste
- *Garnish:* Chopped fresh parsley (optional)

Preparation:

1. Preheat your oven to 400°F (200°C). Then heat your olive oil in a big skillet over medium heat. Add onion and cook until softened, about 5 minutes.

2. Stir in garlic, carrot, and celery. Cook for an additional 2 minutes, or until softened.

3. Add the rinsed lentils, diced tomatoes, veggie broth, thyme, and rosemary. Bring to a boil and cook for 20-25 minutes, or until the lentils are tender. Put salt and pepper to taste.

4. While the lentils cook, make the creamy cashew mash: Drain the soaked cashews and rinse well. In a blender or food processor, add the cashews, plant-based milk, nutritional yeast (if using), salt, and pepper.

5. Blend until smooth and creamy. Add more plant-based milk if needed to achieve the desired consistency.

6. Transfer the lentil filling to a baking dish. Spread the creamy cashew mash on top and allow to bake for 15-20 minutes, or until the top is slightly golden brown.

7. **Serve:** Plate the lentil shepherd's pie and top with chopped fresh parsley (optional).

Nutritional Value (per serving):

- Calories: 400
- Protein: 30g
- Fat: 15g
- Carbohydrates: 40g

Tofu Scramble with Vegetables and Avocado Toast

Ingredients:

Tofu Scramble:

- 1/2 block firm tofu, drained and pressed
- 1/2 tablespoon olive oil
- 1/4 cup chopped onion

- 1/4 cup chopped bell pepper (any color)
- 1/4 cup chopped mushrooms
- 1/4 teaspoon turmeric powder
- 1/4 teaspoon smoked pepper
- Salt and pepper to taste
- Fresh herbs (parsley or chives) for garnish (optional) all chopped

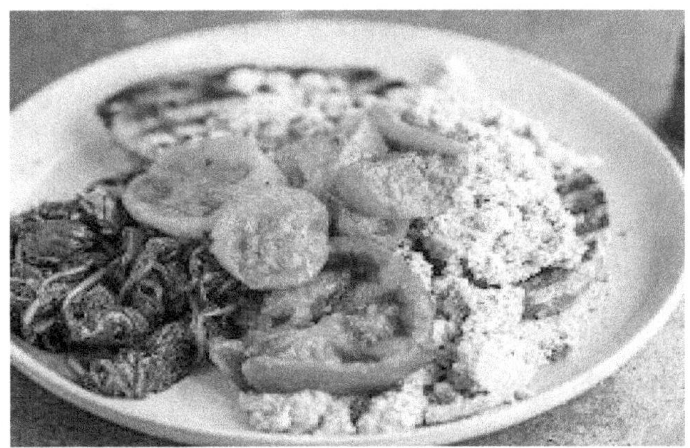

Avocado Toast:

- one slice of whole-wheat bread, toasted
- 1/2 avocado, sliced

- Pinch of lemon juice

Preparation:

1. Crumble the dried and pressed tofu with your hands or a fork. Then heat your olive oil in a pan over medium heat. Put onion and cook until softened, about 3 minutes.

2. Stir in bell pepper and mushrooms, and cook for an additional 2 minutes.

3. Add the broken tofu, turmeric powder, smoked paprika, salt, and pepper. Cook for 5-7 minutes, or until warm through.

4. Toast the whole-wheat bread.

5. While the toast cooks, mash the avocado with a fork and add a squeeze of lemon juice to avoid browning.

6. Spread the mashed avocado on the warm bread.

7. **Serve:** Plate the tofu scramble and top with chopped fresh herbs (optional). Enjoy with the avocado toast.

Nutritional Value (per serving):

- Calories: 400
- Protein: 25g
- Fat: 20g
- Carbohydrates: 35g

Cooking Time 20 minutes

Serving: 1

Edamame and Quinoa Salad with Roasted Vegetables

Ingredients:

Salad:

- 1 cup cooked quinoa

- 1 cup fresh edamame, cooked and cooled
- 1/2 cup chopped cucumber
- 1/4 cup cherry tomatoes, halved
- 1/4 cup crumbled feta cheese (optional)
- 2 tablespoons chopped fresh parsley
- 1 tablespoon olive oil
- 1 tablespoon lemon juice
- Salt and pepper to taste

Roasted Vegetables:

- 1/2 cup broccoli stems
- 1/2 cup chopped bell pepper (any color)
- 1 tablespoon olive oil
- 1/2 teaspoon dried oregano
- Salt and pepper to taste

Preparation:

1. Preheat your oven to 400°F (200°C).

2. ***Roast the vegetables:*** Toss broccoli pieces and chopped bell pepper with olive oil, oregano, salt, and pepper. Stretch them on a baking sheet in a single layer.

3. Roast for 15-20 minutes, or until tender-crisp.

4. While the veggies roast, prepare the salad: In a large bowl, mix cooked quinoa, edamame, chopped cucumber, cherry tomatoes, crumbled feta cheese (if using), and chopped parsley.

5. In another small bowl, mix lemon juice, olive oil, salt, and pepper to form dressing.

6. Assemble the salad: Once the vegetables are roasted, add them to the salad bowl with the other

seasonings. Drizzle with the prepared dressing and toss to mix.

7. *Serve:* Enjoy the edamame and quinoa salad with roasted veggies at room temperature.

Nutritional Value (per serving):

- Calories: 400
- Protein: 25g
- Fat: 18g
- Carbohydrates: 35g

Cooking Time: 30 minutes

Serving: 2

Chickpea Curry with Brown Rice

Ingredients:

Curry:

- 1 tablespoon olive oil

- 1 onion, chopped

- 2 cloves garlic, minced

- 1 tablespoon chopped ginger

- 1 teaspoon curry spice

- 1/2 teaspoon turmeric powder

- Undrained 1 (14.5 oz) can of diced tomatoes

- 1 cup low-sodium veggie broth

- Rinsed and drained one (15 oz) can of chickpeas

- 1/2 cup chopped fresh spinach

- 1/4 cup chopped fresh cilantro

- Salt and pepper to taste

- ***Brown Rice:*** 1/2 cup brown rice, washed

Preparation:

1. Cook the brown rice according to package directions while making the chickpea curry, heat your olive oil in a

big pot or Dutch oven over medium heat. Put onion and cook until softened, about 5 minutes.

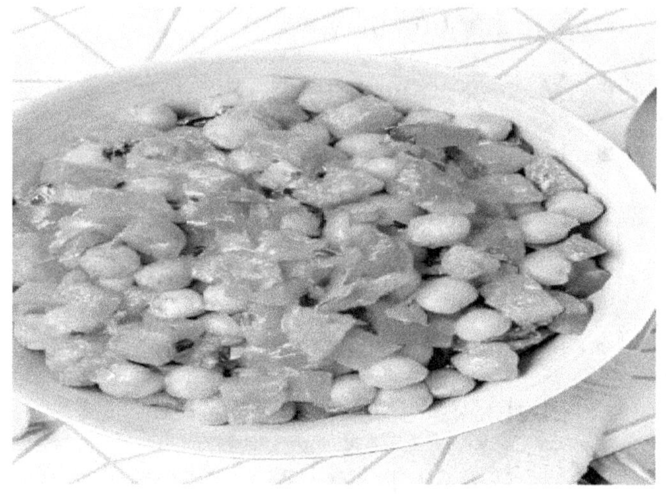

2. Stir in garlic and ginger, and cook for an additional minute, until fragrant.

3. Add curry powder and turmeric powder, and cook for another minute, stirring constantly to release the flavors.

4. Pour in the diced tomatoes and veggie broth. Carry to a boil and cook for 10 minutes.

5. Stir in the drained and rinsed beans and simmer for an additional 10 minutes.

6. Add the chopped spinach and cook for another minute, or until wilted. Then stir in the chopped cilantro and season with salt and pepper to taste.

7. *Serve:* Plate the cooked brown rice and top with the chickpea curry.

Nutritional Value (per serving):

- Calories: 450
- Protein: 30g
- Fat: 10g
- Carbohydrates: 45g

Cooking Time: 40 minutes,

Serving: 2

Ingredients:

Porridge:

- 1/2 cup rolled oats
- 1 cup plain plant-based milk (such as almond or soy milk)
- 1/4 cup water
- 1 tablespoon hemp seeds
- 1/2 teaspoon dried cinnamon
- Pinch of salt

Toppings (optional):

- 1/4 cup fresh berries (such as blueberries, raspberries, or strawberries)
- One tbsp chopped nuts (such as almonds or walnuts)

- 1 tablespoon shredded unsweetened coconut

Preparation:

1. In a small saucepan, mix rolled oats, plant-based milk, water, hemp seeds, cinnamon, and salt. Carry to a simmer over medium heat, stirring occasionally.

2. Reduce heat and cook for 5-7 minutes, or until the oats reach the preferred consistency. If the porridge becomes too thick, add a splash of more water or plant-based milk.

3. ***Prepare toppings (optional):*** Wash and chop fresh berries. Toast nuts lightly in a dry pan, if using.

4. ***Serve:*** Pour the hot porridge into a bowl. Top with fresh berries, chopped

nuts, and shredded coconut (optional).
Enjoy the warmth.

Nutritional Value (per serving):

- Calories: 400
- Protein: 15g
- Fat: 20g
- Carbohydrates: 40g

Cooking Time: 15 minutes

Serving: 1

Peanut Butter and Banana Smoothie with Chia Seeds

Ingredients:

- 1 cup plain plant-based milk (such as almond or soy milk)
- 1/2 cup frozen banana chunks
- 2 tablespoons creamy peanut butter
- 1 tablespoon chia seeds

- 1/2 teaspoon ground cinnamon (optional)
- Pinch of ground ginger (optional)
- Ice cubes (optional)

Preparation:

1. Combine all ingredients (except ice cubes, if using) in a blender. Blend until smooth and creamy.
2. If wanted, add ice cubes for a thicker consistency.
3. *Serve:* Pour the smoothie into a glass and enjoy instantly.

Nutritional Value (per serving):

- Calories: 350
- Protein: 15g
- Fat: 20g
- Carbohydrates: 30g

Cooking Time: 5 minutes

Serving: 1

Sprouted Mung Bean Salad with Tahini Dressing

Ingredients:

Salad:

- 1 cup sprouted mung beans, cleaned and drained
- 1/2 cup chopped cucumber
- 1/4 cup chopped cherry tomatoes
- 1/4 cup chopped red onion
- 1/4 cup crumbled feta cheese (optional)
- 2 tablespoons chopped fresh parsley

Tahini Dressing:

- 2 tablespoons tahini
- 2 tablespoons lemon juice
- 1 tablespoon olive oil
- 1 clove garlic, minced

- Salt and pepper to taste

Preparation:

1. In a large bowl, mix sprouted mung beans, chopped cucumber, cherry tomatoes, red onion, crumbled feta cheese (if using), and chopped parsley.

2. Prepare the tahini dressing: In a small bowl, mix together tahini, lemon juice, olive oil, minced garlic, salt, and pepper.

3. ***Serve:*** Drizzle the tahini dressing over the salad and toss to mix. Enjoy at room temperature.

Nutritional Value (per serving):

- Calories: 350
- Protein: 20g
- Fat: 15g
- Carbohydrates: 30g

Cooking Time:20 minutes

Serving: 2

Quinoa and Black Bean Burgers with Avocado Crema

Ingredients:

Quinoa and Black Bean Burgers:

- 1/2 cup cooked quinoa
- 1 (15 oz) can black beans, cleaned and drained
- 1/2 cup chopped red onion
- 1/4 cup chopped fresh cilantro
- 1 tablespoon breadcrumbs
- 1 tablespoon olive oil
- 1 teaspoon crushed cumin
- 1/2 teaspoon chili spice
- Salt and pepper to taste
- Hamburger buns

Avocado Crema (optional):

- 1/2 avocado, mashed
- 1 tablespoon lime juice
- 1 tablespoon chopped fresh cilantro
- Salt and pepper to taste

Preparation:

1. Preheat your oven to 400°F (200°C).

2. ***To Make black bean burgers:*** In a big bowl, mash half of the black beans with a fork. Combine with cooked quinoa, leftover whole black beans, chopped onion, chopped cilantro, breadcrumbs, olive oil, cumin, chili powder, salt, and pepper. Mix well to mix.

3. Form the mixture into two equal cakes.

4. Heat a lightly oiled pan over medium heat. Cook the quinoa and black bean burgers for 3-4 minutes per side, or

until golden brown and warm through.

5. ***Prepare the avocado cream (optional):*** In a small bowl, mash the avocado with lime juice, chopped cilantro, salt, and pepper.

6. ***Serve:*** Optionally, serve the quinoa and black bean burgers on hamburger buns. Top with avocado cream (optional).

Nutritional Value (per serving):

- Calories: 450
- Protein: 30g
- Fat: 20g
- Carbohydrates: 40g

Cooking Time: 45 minutes

Serving 2

Chapter 6: Soups and stew

Classic Chicken Noodle Soup

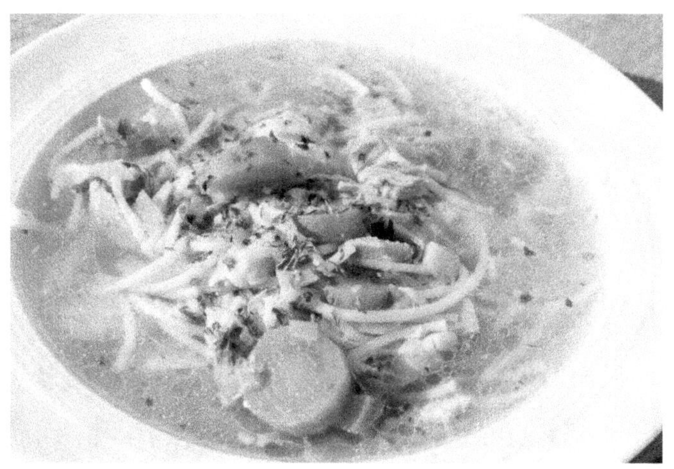

Ingredients:

- 1 tablespoon olive oil
- 1 onion, chopped
- 2 carrots, chopped
- 2 celery stalks, chopped
- 2 cloves garlic, minced
- 8 cups chicken soup

- 1 bay leaf
- 4 skinless and boneless chicken thighs, split or quartered
- 1/2 cup chopped fresh mushrooms (optional)
- 1 cup egg noodles
- Salt and pepper to taste
- Chopped fresh parsley (optional, for garnish)

Preparation:

1. Warm your olive oil in a large pot over medium heat. Put onion, carrots, and celery and cook for 5 minutes, or until softened. Then stir in the garlic and cook for an additional minute, pour in the chicken stock and add the bay leaf. Carry to a boil, reduce heat, and cook for 15 minutes.

2. Add the chicken pieces and onions (optional). Allow to simmer for an additional 20-25 minutes, or until the chicken is cooked through.

3. Remove the bay leaf and cut the cooked chicken with two forks in the pot.

4. Add the egg noodles and cook for another 5 minutes, or until the noodles are soft.

5. Put a little salt and pepper to taste.

6. *Serve:* Ladle the hot soup into bowls and top with chopped fresh parsley (optional).

Nutritional Value per serving:

- Calories: 400
- Protein (30g)
- Fiber: 20
- fat:15

Cooking Time: 1 hour

Serving: 4

<u>Bean & Halloumi Stew</u>

Ingredients:

Base:

- 1 tablespoon olive oil
- 1 onion, chopped
- 1 red bell pepper, chopped
- 2 garlic cloves, minced
- 1 teaspoon dried oregano
- 1/2 teaspoon ground cumin (optional)
- 1 (400g) can chopped tomatoes, undrained
- 400ml vegetable broth
- 1 tablespoon tomato sauce
- 1 bay leaf
- Salt and pepper to taste

Beans & Halloumi:

- 1 (400g) can mixed beans, drained and washed (such as kidney beans, black beans, or chickpeas)
- 1 (400g) can cannellini beans, drained and rinsed
- 250g halloumi cheese, sliced (about 1/2 cm thick)
- 1 tablespoon olive oil (for frying)

Preparation:

1. Heat olive oil in a big pot or Dutch oven over medium heat. Put onion, bell pepper, and garlic and cook for 5 minutes, or until softened.

2. Then stir in oregano, and cumin (optional), and cook for an additional minute, allowing the spices to release their flavor.

3. Add the chopped tomatoes with their juices, veggie broth, tomato paste, and bay leaf. Carry to a boil, reduce heat, and cook for 15 minutes.

4. Stir in the drained and cleaned mixed beans and cannellini beans. Simmer for an extra 10 minutes, allowing the flavors to meld. Put salt and pepper to taste.

5. *Meanwhile:* Heat olive oil in a different frying pan over medium heat. Add the halloumi slices and cook for 2-3 minutes per side or until golden brown and slightly crispy.

6. *Serve:* Ladle the hot stew into bowls and top with the pan-fried halloumi pieces. Remove the bay leaf before serving.

7. ***Optional Additions:*** For a heartier
stew, you can add cooked shredded
chicken or cooked brown rice.

Nutritional Value per serving:

- Calories: 450

- Protein (25g)

- Fiber 10g

Cooking Time: 45 minutes

Serving: 4

Beef Stew with Vegetables

Ingredients:

- 1 tablespoon olive oil

- One pound of beef stew meat cut into
  bite-sized pieces

- 1 onion, chopped

- 2 carrots, chopped

- 2 celery stalks, chopped

- 2 cloves garlic, minced
- 1 tablespoon tomato sauce
- 1 teaspoon dried thyme
- 1/2 teaspoon dried rosemary
- 1 bay leaf
- 4 cups beef broth
- 1 cup red wine (optional)
- Undrained 1 (14.5 oz) can of diced tomatoes
- 1/2 cup frozen peas
- Salt and pepper to taste
- Chopped fresh parsley (optional, for garnish)

Preparation:

1. Warm your olive oil in a large Dutch oven or pot over medium-high heat and sear the beef stew meat in batches until cooked on all sides. Remove the

cooked meat from the pot and set aside.

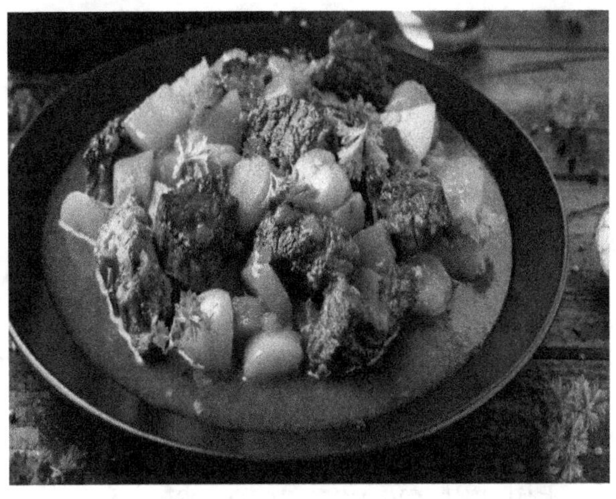

2. In the same pot, add carrots, onion, and celery and cook for 5 minutes, or until softened.

3. Stir in the garlic, tomato paste, thyme, rosemary, and bay leaf. Cook for an extra minute, allowing the spices to release their aroma.

4. Add the cooked beef pieces back to the pot along with the beef broth, red

wine (optional), and diced tomatoes with their juices.

5. Carry to a boil, then reduce heat, cover the pot, and simmer for 1-1.5 hours, or until the beef is soft and falling off the bone.

6. About 15 minutes before the stew is finished cooking, stir in the frozen peas.

7. Put salt and pepper to taste.

8. *Serve:* Ladle the hot stew into bowls and top with chopped fresh parsley (optional).

Nutritional value per serving:

- Calories: 500
- Protein (40g)

Cooking Time: 1.5 hours

Serves: 4

Creamy Mushroom Soup

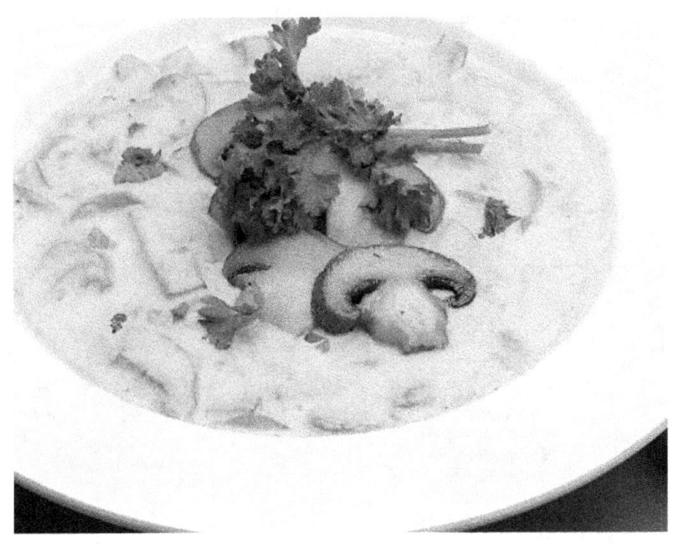

Ingredients:

- 1 tablespoon olive oil

- 1 onion, chopped

- 2 cloves garlic, minced

- 1 pound mixed mushrooms, sliced (such as cremini, portobello, shiitake)

- 1/2 teaspoon dried thyme

- 4 cups vegetable broth

- 1 cup heavy cream (or low-fat cream for a lighter version)
- 1/4 cup grated Parmesan cheese
- Salt and pepper to taste
- 1/4 cup cooked shredded chicken or cooked broken tofu (optional, for a protein boost)
- Chopped fresh parsley (optional, for garnish)

Preparation:

1. Heat olive oil in a big pot or Dutch oven over medium heat. Put onion and garlic and cook for 5 minutes, or until softened.

2. Stir in the chopped mushrooms and thyme. Cook for an additional 5 minutes, or until the mushrooms are softened and release their juices.

3. Put your veggie broth and carry it to a boil. Minimize heat and simmer for 10 minutes.

4. Using an immersion blender or a blender in batches, puree the soup until smooth and rich. (For a chunkier soup, leave some mushrooms unblended)

5. Stir in the heavy cream and Parmesan cheese. Put salt and pepper to taste.

6. Heat through for a few minutes longer.

7. *Serve:* Ladle the hot soup into bowls. Top with cooked shredded chicken or crumbled tofu (optional) and serve with chopped fresh parsley (optional).

Nutritional Value per serving:

- *Calories: 350 per serving (without protein boost) / 400 per serving (with chicken) / 300 per serving (with tofu)*
- *Key Nutrients: Protein (15g without protein boost / 25g with chicken / 20g with tofu), Vitamin D (from mushrooms), Calcium (from Parmesan cheese)*

Cooking Time: 30 minutes
Serving: 4

Somerset Stew with Cheddar & Parsley Mash

Ingredients:
Stew:

- 1 tablespoon vegetable oil
- 1 onion, chopped
- 2 carrots, diced
- 2 garlic cloves, minced

- 1 tablespoon tomato purée

- 400g can chopped tomatoes

- 200g can butter beans, drained

- 400g can flageolet beans, rinsed and drained

- 250ml dry cider (or replace with chicken broth)

- 250ml vegetable stock

- Few sprigs of fresh thyme, leaves only

- Salt and pepper to taste

Cheddar & Parsley Mash:

- 850g potatoes, sliced and cut into chunks

- 25g butter

- 75g extra-mature cheddar cheese, grated

- Handful of fresh parsley, chopped

- Milk (optional, for changing mash consistency)
- Salt and pepper to taste

Preparation:

1. ***Stew:*** Heat the vegetable oil in a big pot or Dutch oven over medium heat. Put chopped onion and diced carrots and cook for 5 minutes, or until softened.
2. Stir in the chopped garlic and tomato purée. Then cook for an additional minute, allowing the flavors to blend.
3. Add the chopped tomatoes, drained butter beans, rinsed and drained flageolet beans, cider (or broth), and veggie stock.
4. Bring to a boil, then reduce heat and simmer for 30 minutes, or until the

veggies are tender and the stew has thickened slightly.

5. Season with salt and pepper to taste. Remove the thyme leaves from the sprigs and discard the stems (optional).

6. ***Cheddar & Parsley Mash:*** While the stew simmers, bring a big pot of salted water to a boil. Add the cubed potatoes and cook for 15-20 minutes, or until tender when poked with a fork. Then drain the potatoes well and return them to the pot. Crush the potatoes with a potato masher or use a hand mixer for a smoother consistency.

7. Add the butter, grated cheddar cheese, and chopped fresh parsley. Put salt and pepper to taste.

8. If the mash seems too dry, add a splash of milk at a time until you hit the desired consistency.

9. *Serve:* Ladle the hot stew into bowls and top with large scoops of the creamy cheddar and parsley mash. Enjoy!

Nutritional Value per serving:

- Calories: 500
- Protein (25g)

Cooking Time: 1 hour 15 minutes

Serving: 4

Chapter 7: High protein Snacks and Appetizer

Edamame with a Twist

Ingredients:

- 1 cup frozen shelled edamame
- 1/2 teaspoon olive oil
- Pinch of garlic powder
- Pinch of chili flakes (adjust for spice taste)
- Pinch of sea salt

Preparation:

1. Microwave the frozen edamame according to package guidelines until heated through.
2. While hot, toss the edamame with olive oil, garlic powder, chili flakes (optional), and sea salt.

3. Serve: Enjoy the edamame warm or at
   room temperature.

Nutritional value:

- Protein (17g)
- Fiber (8g)

Cooking Time: 5 minutes

Serving: 1

Cottage Cheese Scramble with Vegetables

Ingredients:

- 1/2 cup low-fat cottage cheese
- 1/4 cup chopped bell pepper
- 1/4 cup chopped mushrooms
- 1 tablespoon chopped chives
- 1 egg, beaten
- Salt and pepper to taste

Preparation:

1. Heat a small non-stick pan over medium heat. with non-stick cooking oil.

2. Sauté the chopped bell pepper and mushrooms until softened.

3. In a different bowl, whisk together cottage cheese and beaten egg.

4. Pour the cottage cheese mixture into the pan with the veggies. Scramble with a spoon until cooked through.

5. Season with salt, pepper, and chopped chives.

6. Serve: Enjoy the cottage cheese stir hot or at room temperature.

Nutritional Value:

- Protein (18g)

Cooking Time: 15 minutes

Serving: 1

Ingredients:

- 1 pound lean ground turkey
- 1/2 cup chopped onion
- 1/4 cup chopped bell pepper
- 1/4 cup chopped carrot
- 1/4 cup rolled oats
- 1 egg, beaten
- 1 tablespoon ketchup
- 1 tablespoon Worcestershire sauce
- 1/2 teaspoon dried thyme
- Salt and pepper to taste

Preparation:

1. Preheat your oven to 375°F (190°C). Grease a 12-cup muffin pan.

2. In a large bowl, mix ground turkey, chopped onion, bell pepper, carrot, rolled oats, beaten egg, ketchup,

Worcestershire sauce, thyme, salt, and pepper. Mix well.

3. Divide the mixture equally among the prepared muffin tins and bake for 20-25 minutes, or until cooked through.

4. *Serve:* Let the muffins cool slightly before serving. You can enjoy them warm or at room temperature.

Nutritional Value:

- Protein: 20g

Cooking Time: 45 minutes

makes 12 muffins

Hard-boiled egg with Avocado & Chia Seed Toast

Ingredients:

- 1 slice whole-wheat bread, toasted
- 1/2 avocado, mashed

- 1 hard-boiled egg, sliced

- 1 tablespoon lemon juice (optional)

- 1 tablespoon chia seeds

- Salt and pepper to taste

Preparation:

1. Toast a slice of whole-wheat bread.

2. Spread mashed avocado on the toast.

3. Top with sliced hard-boiled egg.

4. Drizzle with lemon juice (optional).

5. Sprinkle chia seeds and season with salt and pepper to taste.

Nutritional value:

- Protein (6g from egg)

Cooking Time: 10 minutes

Serving: 1

Tuna Salad on Cucumber Slices

Ingredients:

- Drained 1 can (5 oz) canned tuna in water

- 1 tablespoon mayonnaise (or light mayonnaise)

- 1 tablespoon chopped celery (optional)

- 1/4 teaspoon dried dill

- Salt and pepper to taste

- 1 big cucumber, sliced

Preparation:

1. In a bowl, mix flaked tuna, mayonnaise, chopped celery (optional), dried dill, salt, and pepper. Mix well.

2. Wash and slice a big cucumber into rounds or sticks.

3. Serve: Top the cucumber pieces with the tuna salad mixture. Enjoy this snack cold.

- Protein: 20g from tuna)

Preparation Time: 5 minutes
Servind: 1

Cottage Cheese with Sliced Apple and Cinnamon

Ingredients:

- 1/2 cup low-fat cottage cheese
- 1 small apple, diced
- 1/2 teaspoon dried cinnamon
- Honey drizzle (optional)

Preparation:

1. Put the cottage cheese in a bowl.
2. Top with sliced apple.
3. Sprinkle it with ground cinnamon.
4. Drizzle with honey for additional taste (optional).

Nutritional Value:

Protein: 18g from cottage cheese)

Preparation Time: 5 minutes

Serving 1

Conclusion

In the culinary journey described in the "High-Protein Cookbook for Seniors," we've explored the transformative power of nutrition tailored especially for the golden years. As we finish this culinary guide, it's clear that food isn't merely sustenance; it's a key ally in promoting vibrant health and vitality among seniors.

Through a careful selection of high-protein ingredients and thoughtful meal planning, this cookbook wants to empower seniors to take charge of their well-being. You have found the importance of protein-rich diets in preserving muscle mass, supporting bone health, and addressing common health concerns. The recipes provided are not just delicious; they are a celebration of life, giving a diverse array of flavors and nutrients to meet the unique nutritional needs of seniors.

From grilled chicken salads to nutrient-packed quinoa bowls, each recipe is created to balance protein with essential vitamins, minerals, and fiber. The incorporation of lean meats, poultry, fish, and plant-based protein sources provides a complete approach to senior nutrition.

As we bid farewell to the pages of this cookbook, let it be a lesson that aging doesn't mean compromising on flavor or nutrition. Rather, it's a chance to embrace a high-protein lifestyle that nourishes the body, uplifts the spirit, and adds to a fulfilling and active senior life. May these recipes not only tantalize the taste buds but also inspire a renewed dedication to health and wellness among our beloved seniors.

Cheers to a future filled with good food, good health, and the joy of enjoying life's flavors to the fullest.

www.ingramcontent.com/pod-product-compliance
Lightning Source LLC
Chambersburg PA
CBHW051553250726
48653CB00004BA/1127